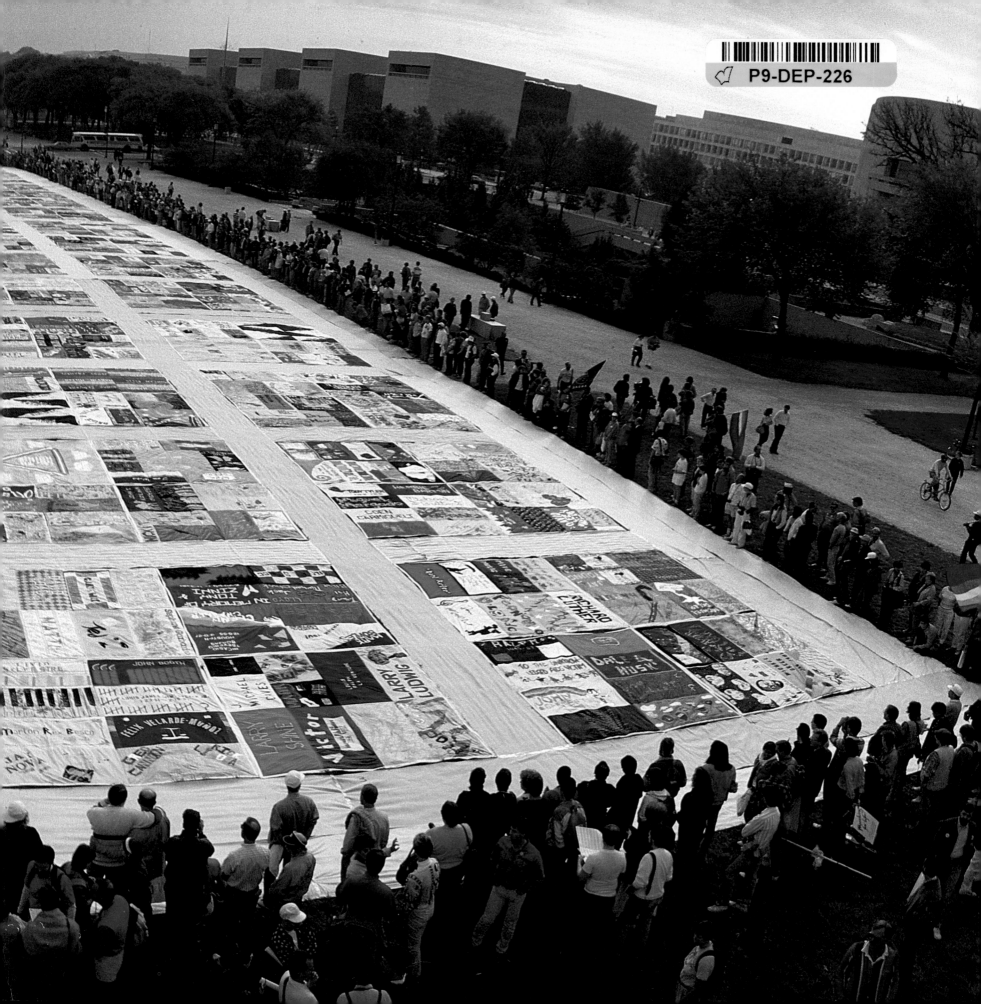

THE
QUILT

Stories From
The NAMES Project

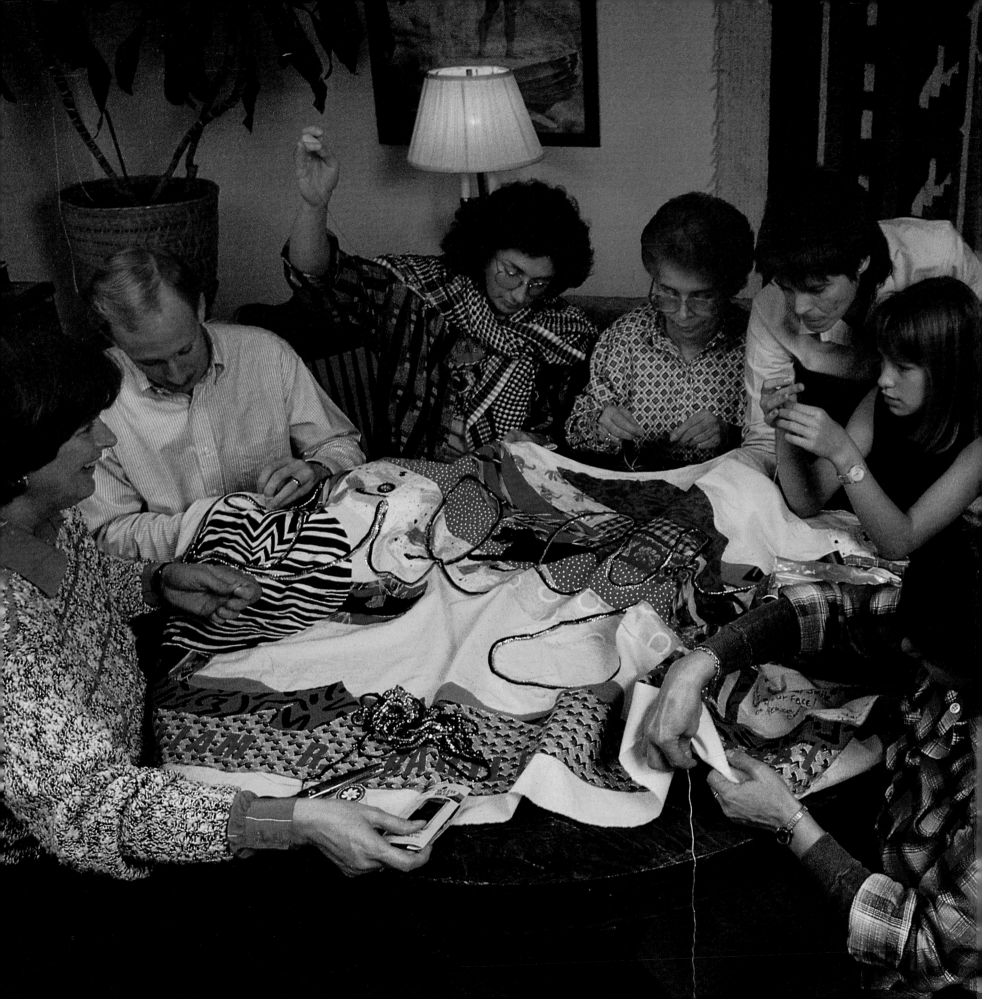

THE QUILT

Stories From
The NAMES Project

Written by Cindy Ruskin
Photographs by Matt Herron
Design by Deborah Zemke

With an introduction by Elizabeth Taylor

POCKET BOOKS

New York   London   Toronto   Sydney   Tokyo

Another *Original* publication of POCKET BOOKS

POCKET BOOKS, a division of Simon & Schuster, Inc.
1230 Avenue of the Americas, New York, N.Y. 10020

ISBN: 0–671–66597–9

First Pocket Books trade hardcover printing May, 1988

10 9 8 7 6 5 4 3 2 1

POCKET and colophon are trademarks of Simon & Schuster, Inc.

Printed in the U.S.A.

To the people we have come to know through the quilt panels they have made, and for those we know through the panels made for them. We also dedicate this book to the 25,000 Americans not named in The Quilt who have died of AIDS, and to the families, lovers and friends who miss them.

The NAMES Project

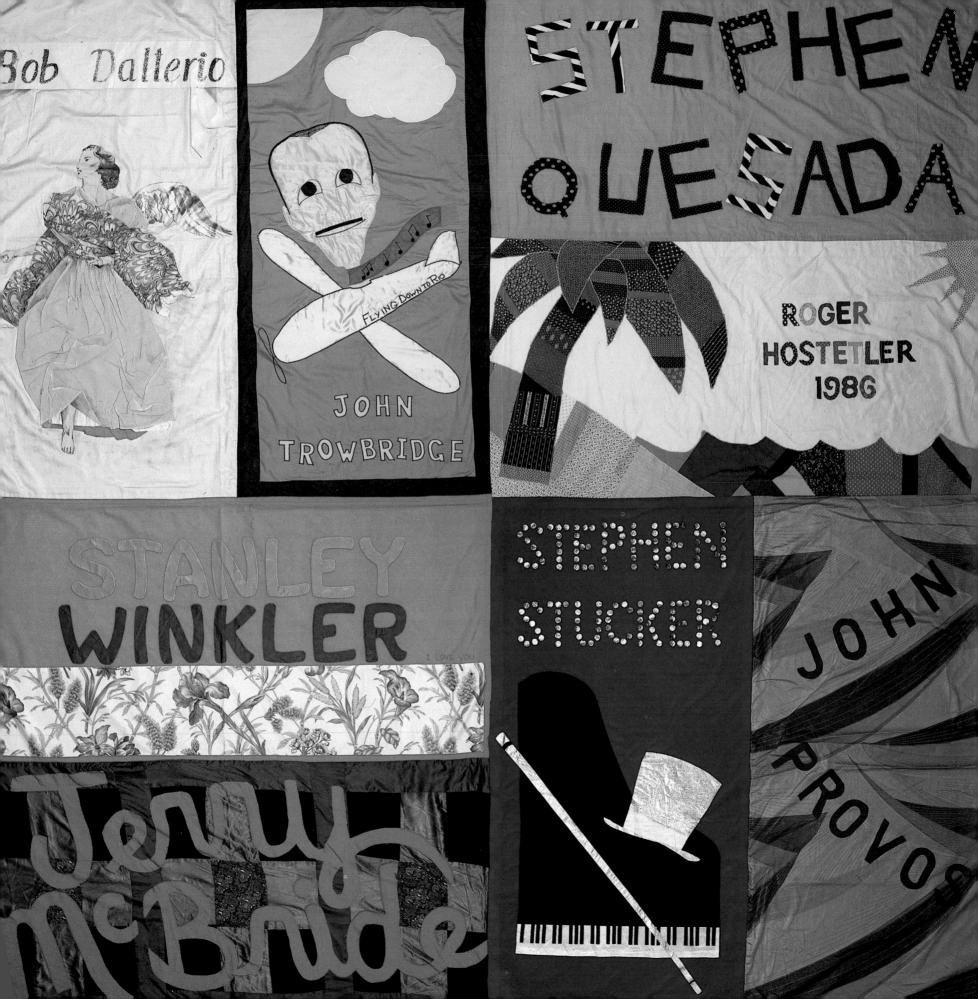

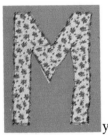y grandparents, well into their eighties, grow melancholy remembering lifelong friends who have died. At thirty-four, I know how they feel." These words were written by a young man several years ago about his feelings upon losing so many loved ones to AIDS.

AIDS has come upon us with cruel abandon. It has forced us to confront and deal with the frailty of our being and the reality of death. It has forced us into a realization that we must cherish every moment of the glorious experience of this thing we call life. We are learning to value our own lives and the lives of our loved ones as if any moment may be the last.

Many of us have lost loved ones to AIDS. We grieve. We suffer the seemingly endless pain. We bear the emptiness that yearns to be filled. We strive to find meaning in the fact that someone so dear has left us. We search for lessons to learn. We remember the joy, passion and sensitive interconnections which filled our relationships.

We fight in the face of obstacles that seem insurmountable. We endure because we must. We comfort those in need because we care. We renew our efforts daily, in the face of this nightmare that is real.

We rise and fall, and rise again to meet the challenge of AIDS. As Americans, we have always risen to meet the most difficult of challenges. And in the historic tradition of compassion and caring, hard work and commitment, and perseverance, we will continue to rise to meet the challenge.

The Quilt is a moving depiction of stories of the loved ones of human beings who have died of AIDS. It reflects the true spirit of America. In their tragedy and grief over loss immeasurable, contributors to The Quilt have used art and love to keep the spirit of their loved ones alive.

People with AIDS and AIDS-related conditions confront ultimate challenges. Their supreme courage in their personal fight against AIDS has set standards for all of us to follow. Their loved ones have shared in this challenge and have demonstrated similar courage. *The Quilt* relates stories of such courage.

The Quilt gives us our most direct feelings back; our feelings of belonging, our sense of the precariousness of life, why it is worth clinging to, how it can be lived, how tragically it can be lost, how beautifully, after all, it can be relinquished, and how vibrantly it can be remembered.

As Americans touched by the AIDS crisis, we must rise above our personal considerations and open our hearts to those in need. We must offer genuine expressions of our love and caring, in whatever form is possible.

In the common bond of humanity, we are all one. We all possess the basic desires of wanting love and wanting to love. We all share experiences of love, pain, joy, sadness, anger, and exhilaration.

After reading this book, you will possess a deeper sense of yourself and a deeper sense of your kind — the human community of life and death, of shared joy and suffering. *The Quilt* is a masterpiece created out of love by The NAMES Project. It is a rare and intense experience of what it means to be human.

Elizabeth Taylor

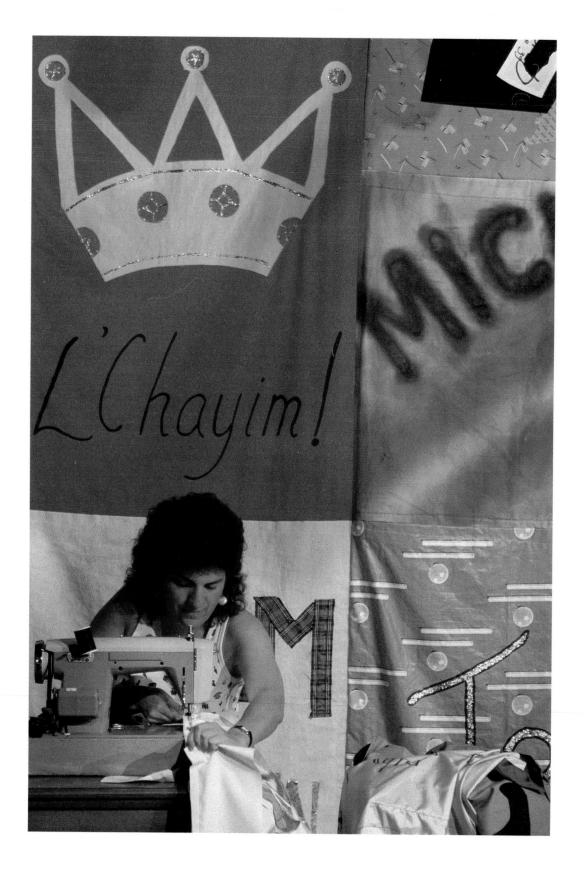

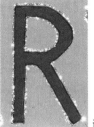icky Riccobono really was one of the great kind souls of the earth," writes a friend. "No, you probably won't recognize his name. He never appeared on the cover of *Time*, never had dinner at the White House, and didn't even have a rotary club luncheon in his honor. All he had, which made him a very wealthy man, was the deep, abiding love of many, many dear friends." In January 1987, Ricky Riccobono died of AIDS.

After dinner one night, two of his friends sat around a dining room table in Barre, Vermont, to make a cloth memorial, spelling out Ricky's name with colored markers in a cross-stitch design. When it was done, the fabric banner was mailed off to The NAMES Project in San Francisco's Castro district. There it joined 3,000 other panels being sewn together in one enormous quilt. Like Ricky's, each of these quilt panels bears the name of someone who has died of AIDS; and also like Ricky's, each embodies the love and grief of the family, friends and lovers who created it.

The NAMES Project is a national effort to create a hand-sewn tribute to the tens of thousands of Americans stricken down by AIDS. The idea for the Project originated the night of November 27, 1985, when San Francisco activist Cleve Jones joined several thousand others in the annual candlelight march commemorating the murders of Mayor George Moscone and Harvey Milk, San Francisco's first openly gay supervisor. As the mourners passed by, they covered the walls of San Francisco's old Federal Building with placards bearing the names of people who had died of AIDS. "It was such a startling image," remembers Cleve. "The wind and the rain tore some of the cardboard names loose, but people stood there for hours reading names. I knew then that we needed a monument, a memorial."

That image of cardboard placards eventually gave way to the vision of a unifying quilt in memory of those who had died of AIDS. "Let's take all of our individual experiences," Cleve thought, "and stitch them together to make something that has strength and beauty."

The Quilt idea took off a year later, in the spring of 1987, when Cleve teamed up with Mike Smith, 27, a recent graduate of Stanford Business School. Together they organized local sewing bees — small groups of friends gathered in San Francisco apartments — and on June 28, the still-fledgling NAMES Project displayed its first 40 panels at San Francisco's Lesbian and Gay Freedom Day Parade, hanging them from the mayor's balcony at City Hall. Cleve Jones and Mike Smith then told AIDS resource organizations across the country that The NAMES Project was

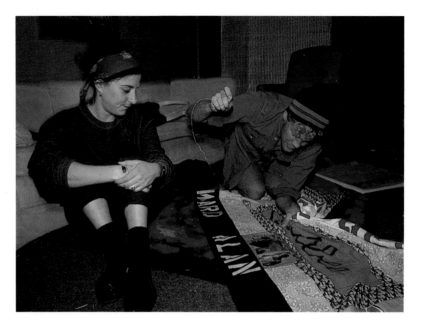

under way, and they began planning for a giant quilt for display in Washington, D.C., during October's National March for Lesbian and Gay Rights.

By mid-July, as quilt panels were piling up on Mike Smith's back porch, he searched for a workshop to store and assemble them. The NAMES Project found a home in an empty Market Street storefront in the Castro, San Francisco's main gay neighborhood. There, Cleve, Mike, and the Project's technical director, Ron Cordova, set up what was then a shoestring operation. "We thought that we had so much space," recalls a laughing Mike, looking around the now-jammed headquarters. "It felt like a huge cavern."

While seven volunteers shared the Project's single borrowed sewing machine in a room that was initially without lights, Cleve taped a sheet of butcher paper outside the front door with the announcement: "This is the new home of The NAMES Project and this is our wish list. . . ." They needed everything from sequins, beads, fabric and glue to extension cords, computers, telephones, lights and furniture. At the end of the list, Cleve added "back rubs, hugs and money."

The Castro was quick in responding to The NAMES Project's call. Within two weeks, The Project had received ten sewing machines, including three industrial models, and the storefront

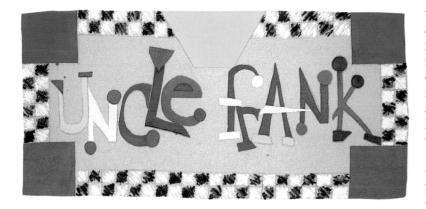

was flooded with volunteers. "This could not have happened anywhere else in the country," says Mike. "There is no other neighborhood that has been so affected by the disease. There is no other neighborhood that has been so generous." Local merchants paid $2000 for the Project's first month's rent. The storefront's previous tenants provided track lighting. Someone left an anonymous gift of $500 in the donation box. A chiropractor regularly donated full body massages until midnight for volunteers who spent the day doubled over sewing machines.

The volunteers' primary task is sewing together eight individual three-by-six-foot panels into larger quilt sections measuring 12 feet square. The job was manageable at first, as only 400 panels had arrived by late August. But during the first weeks of September, hundreds of bundles began to arrive, often by Federal Express to meet the deadline for the Washington, D.C. unveiling. By early October, the shelves in the Market Street storefront overflowed with needles, bobbins, thread and yet-to-be-stitched panels, as volunteers worked around the clock to put together as many of the late arrivals as they could. Ultimately, 1,920 quilt panels made it to the Capitol Mall in Washington, where they covered an area the size of two football fields. But nearly 3,000 panels had reached the San Francisco workshop by the time of the March and they haven't stopped coming.

The NAMES Project remains a center of bustling activity in the Castro, as panels continue to arrive and The Quilt embarks on a nationwide tour to raise funds for AIDS-related services such as hospices, food delivery programs and in-home support services. Six staffers, 25 full-time volunteers and hundreds of part-timers work day and night to sew hems, stitch panels, and attach the grommets that will join the quilts to white fabric walkways. Some people spend weeks at The NAMES Project workshop creating a quilt panel, and occasionally volunteers are commissioned to make a panel for someone who is unable to do it.

Project volunteers are often called upon to make alterations and rescue troubled panels. Many quilters are learning to use a sewing machine for the first time. A note from one novice apologetically explains that the panel is the wrong size because it shrank in the wash. "I felt that it would be best to leave it to you all to sew a straight line," says Maurice Higdon of Portland, who marked the three-inch hem margin with a pink pencil "rather than botch up, making it so that you all had to rip it out and resew it." Higdon borrowed a sewing machine, broke the needle, jammed the arm, and stayed up till 3 A.M. working on the panel for his lover. Another hapless tailor wrote to The NAMES Project, "It didn't turn out exactly as I envisioned, but I'm not exactly Betsy Ross."

The Project is a place not only of hard work but of strong emotions. Every day someone walking by recognizes a name written on a panel, learning for the first time that a friend has died. A young man with AIDS comes in to make his own panel. A woman breaks down in tears as she hands over the memorial

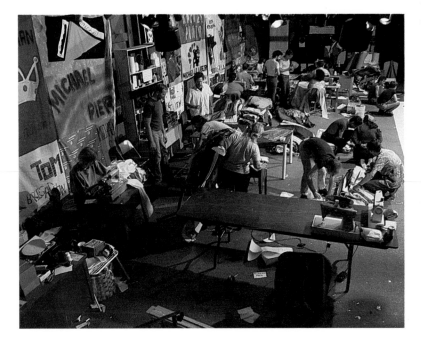

that she made for a close friend. Project volunteers with AIDS-related illnesses disappear when they become too sick to leave their homes.

But if The NAMES Project frequently brings home the painful reality of AIDS, it also provides a place of sharing and comfort. Gini Spiersch, 44, a mother of two, volunteered at The NAMES Project after 11 of her coworkers at a gay-owned record company died within a few years. "The most devastating thing you can put on a panel is a birth date and death date," she says. "They're so young. My boss was 29. In your lifetime, you think you will have to bury a relative, a friend, or maybe there will be a freak accident. Who the hell would think that you'd go to 15 funerals in 19 months?" But Spiersch finds solace in her NAMES Project work. "When you reflect on someone's life," she says, "some of their creativity comes out in the panel. It feels good to know that this person's name will be out there forever."

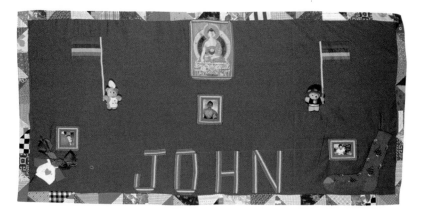

Nancy Katz, 31, discovered The NAMES Project when she walked in to get change for her parking meter. Katz, who teaches quilting at a women's jail, had never known anyone who had died of AIDS, but the panels hanging on the workshop walls had an immediate impact. "I got tearful, blown away as soon as I saw this place," she says. "I just knew that I had to come back. The whole point of quilting is to have a sense of community, and it was important for me to be identified as an ally. It's festive — kind of like being at a summer camp. But it also brings people together to deal with their grief."

"This is a magical place," Cleve says, standing amidst the hubbub of the workshop. "What you see is an extraordinary investment of love, creative energy, and hours and hours of work. There hasn't been a day that I've been there that I haven't cried. But the miracle of that place is that over the sound of sewing machines, you hear the sound of laughter all day long."

As their letters show, thousands of people who have never been to The NAMES Project workshop have been equally affected by The Quilt. Tucked in the packages with the quilt panels are diaries, letters, poems and photographs telling stories of poignant love and loss. One quilt arrived with a full-length play, another with an angry letter addressed directly to God.

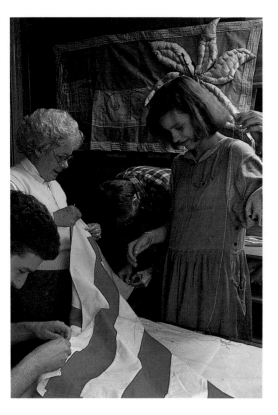

David Taggart's mother remembers the inquisitive little boy who took apart all his toys, the adolescent who started a fire in his bedroom trying to smelt metal, and the teenager who, while backpacking in Madrid, bought a suit of armor in his size. One man fondly recalls the way his lover used to slurp oysters, and the time he cleaned his closet dressed only in a T-shirt, one sock and a pair of headphones. A mother and father look back to the time their son Mark flooded the living room with a whole keg of beer. "We thought that a little beer on the carpet was a tragedy," they write. "Where were our priorities then?"

By the end of 1988, Cleve expects that as many as 10,000 will have made such memories a part of The NAMES Project quilt. One letter in particular affirms his faith in the project's worth. "I

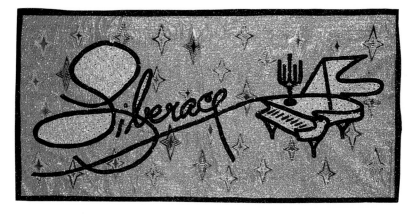

After seeing Liberace in concert in Sioux Falls, South Dakota, 25 years ago, Hollywood designer Warren Caton decided to move to Los Angeles. "He had such a personal effect on my life," says Warren, who wrote on the back of this NAMES Project tribute: "In memory of Liberace, Mr. Showmanship. He showed me that there was a place in the world for more glitz! He made the world brighter and now the heavens have more sparkle."

am so proud to include my son's name among all the others, the brave, dear victims of this dreadful disease," writes a mother. "It will be such a comfort to me and all of us who grieve for them to know that their deaths now will serve a very useful purpose in bringing attention to *all* Americans, and all the world, the enormity of this catastrophe."

Cleve's eyes still glisten, with both sadness and pride, as he reads such a letter. "The Quilt shows that the most important thing is to love and be loved," he says. "Each letter breaks my heart."

This potential for expressions of love and compassion were central to Cleve's idea of a quilt as the form for this AIDS memorial. "By providing a glimpse of the lives behind the statistics," he states, "it will create an extraordinary, dramatic illustration of the magnitude of this epidemic — to the president, to Congress, and to the country. Also, it's a way for survivors to work through their grief in a positive, creative way. Quilts represent coziness, humanity and warmth." For centuries, women have exchanged quilts for friendship, bridal or bereavement purposes. "We want to create something that is beautiful," Cleve says. "The Quilt touches something in people that is pure and good — this is how the country should respond to the AIDS epidemic."

Traditionally, quilts are collaborative works that include a vast array of colors and patterns, and the AIDS Quilt specifically speaks to the diversity of lives affected by the disease. Although the remembrances sewn into each quilt panel can only hint at the person's life, and although the entire quilt records only about 10 percent of the nation's AIDS deaths, the disease's undiscriminating nature is easily seen in the range of the people memorialized. They include a Colorado stockbroker, a mother of four teenagers in Atlanta, an Olympic athlete, a prize-winning Chicago journalist, a biker from Nevada, and a Stanford University professor. Some quilt panels name celebrities like Rock Hudson and Liberace. Others name people who were living on welfare, struggling to keep off the streets. There are policemen, schoolteachers, farmers, doctors, playwrights, ministers, chefs, lawyers, artists and politicians. There is a quilt panel for the hairdresser who styled Joan Mondale's hair during the 1984 Democratic Convention, and there is one for the respiratory therapist who tended Ronald Reagan after the 1981 assassination attempt. There are sons and daughters, mothers and fathers, lovers, brothers, friends and grandparents.

This diversity and individuality are similarly reflected in the panels themselves. Whether drawn, painted, appliquéd or stitched, the quilt panels are spectacularly varied in style, materials and sensibility. Humble little stick figures in crayon and the unsteady handwriting of a child are sewn to stunning, sophisticated renditions by a professional artist. Materials ranging from gold lamé, imported silk and Brooks Brothers tweed to denim, polyester and black leather strive to create a true sense of the person remembered. Names are spelled out in heavy braided

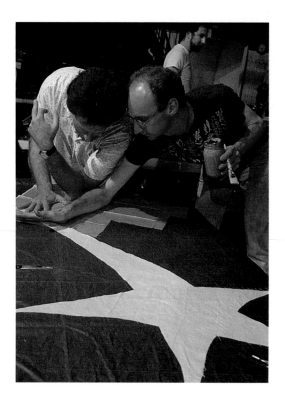

cord, in shiny vinyl cutouts, in zippers, sequins, bits of bright ribbon, glass beads and, of course, glitter galore.

Some panels are literally laden with mementos, possessions and final farewells. Families and friends have rummaged through old belongings, pulling photographs, clothes, Halloween costumes, university pennants, feather boas and military medals to create their quilted scrapbooks. Everything is sewn in: locks of hair, record albums, souvenir postcards, a Barbie doll, whistles, crystals, tuxedos, a shard of glass, giant foam rubber french fries, toy cars on a painted street, a thimble, a giant cowboy hat stuffed with T-shirts to keep its shape, teddy bears, a pink Lacoste shirt, a Buddhist's saffron robe, and even a padded jockstrap. Five panels incorporate the ashes of the people they honor in the design. Impulsively scribbled notes are left in the corners; others are tucked in pockets sewn to the back of quilt panels. In a panel called "Jac from Sac," friends each wrote a private message, now permanently sewn up in a huge bushy mustache. Designer Alan Falconer's panel is a transparent plastic sheet with six Ziploc bags filled with color xeroxes of his own art. "The little heart-shaped pillow is stuffed with my hair," writes Robert Meslinsky of the panel he made for hairdresser Michael Thimmes, "for him to rest his weary head."

The mood of the quilt panels likewise range from the spiritual to the irreverent. Dáhn van Laarz meticulously wrote out his lover's creed of tolerance, creating a panel that is sober and reflective. The panel for Herb Finger expresses rage: bloodlike slashes of red paint drip from his crimson name. Some panels incorporate images of angels and allusions to afterlife reunions. Others opt for whimsy. "Is this Art? No! It's Fred Abrams!" declares the panel of Fred with his red high-heeled legs kicked up on a file cabinet. Even more unabashed is the campy panel for David Kreamer adorned with a red feather boa and the inscription, "Oh he did like to dress up."

Ultimately, each quilt panel has its own tale, and it is the richness, humanity and vital nature of these many and varied stories that together compose the greater story of The NAMES Project. These are not stories of an illness. Rather, they are stories of courage, fear, and anger, and mostly, they are stories of love. They tell of people who worked and played, who laughed and fought, and who are finally remembered.

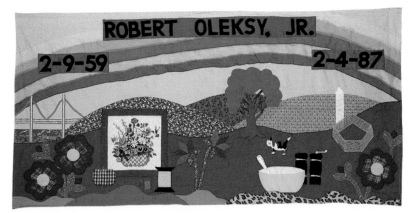

Bobby Oleksy's mother volunteers at Center Project, Inc., an AIDS Resource Center in Wisconsin, helping families through the trauma of having a family member with AIDS. Using Bobby's own needlework, the volunteers at Center Project created this panel to honor Bobby and his mother. Volunteer Gordon Case meticulously stitched the panel, changing the thread to match each different-colored piece of fabric.

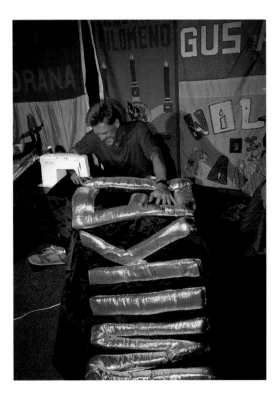

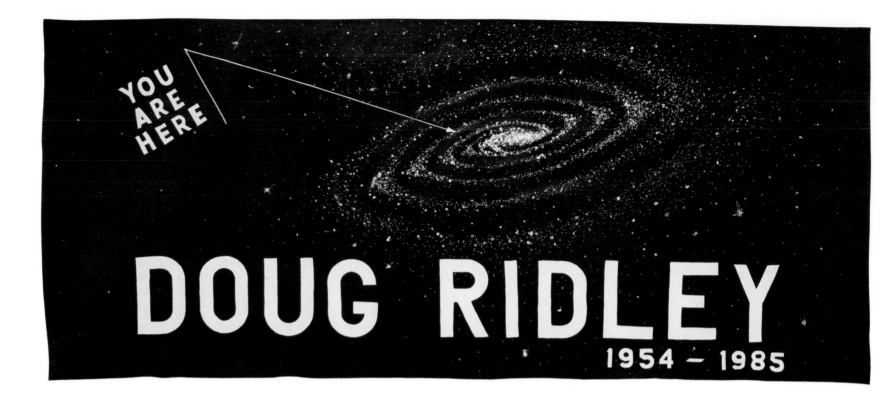

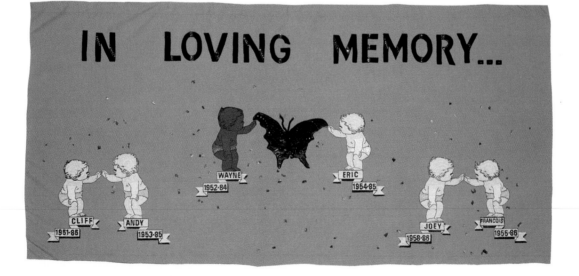

14

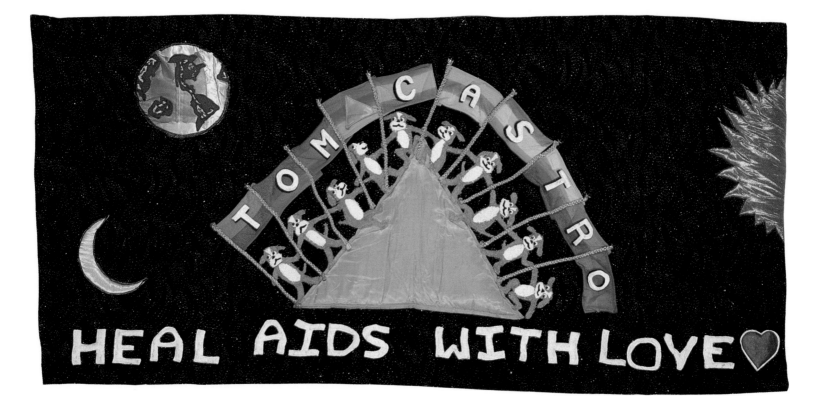

HEAL AIDS WITH LOVE♡

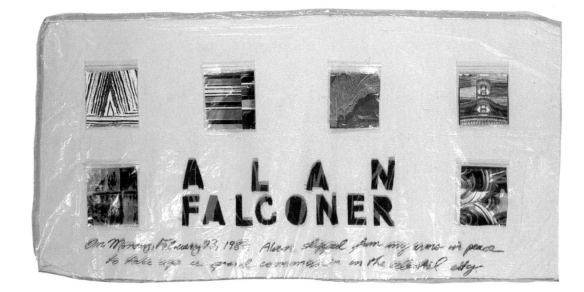

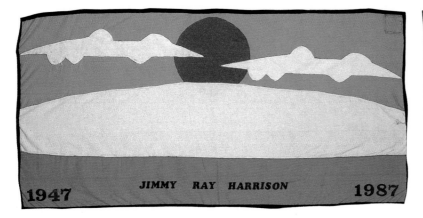

1947   JIMMY RAY HARRISON   1987

Jimmy Harrison lived with AIDS for four years. He died two weeks before his 30th birthday with his lover Jesse Barrenda at his side. Their friend James Finch sewed Jimmy's ashes into the small pocket on the upper right corner of his commemorative panel.

MICHAEL SKLAR

GEORGE • MORRIS • STEVEN • JOE • JIMMY • HARRY • VINCENT • WOODY • ROCK • MICHAEL • LIBERACE • CHARLES • PERRY • WAY • BOB • RICHARD

Four friends created this tribute for actor/businessman Michael Sklar. Michael starred in three Andy Warhol movies and appeared in the revival of "Laugh-In" with Robin Williams. He also founded Child Star, a jewelry and greeting card company in Los Angeles.

16

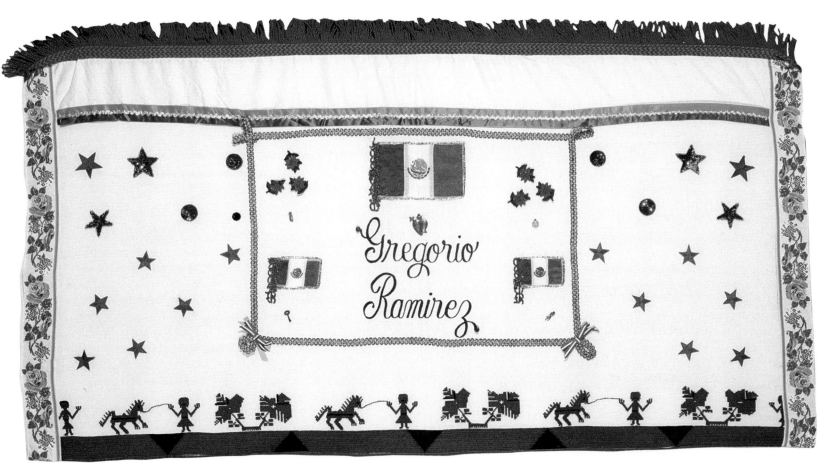

All the decorations on the panel Adriana Williams made to honor Gregorio Ramirez are from Mexico. Adriana knew the young Mexican artist and his family for over 15 years.

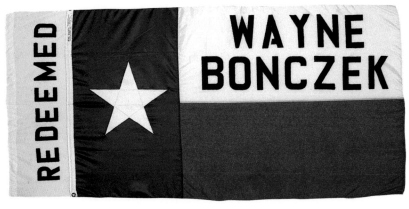

This memorial for Wayne Bonczek was fashioned from a Texan flag.

17

It's one of the strange but wonderful things that happens in a disaster like a plague or a war. All at once a whole nation faces a challenge — the challenge to be there for one another and to help each other through. There's nothing good about this plague, but there's a lot of good in the way people respond to it. What we're trying to do in the Project is to touch people's hearts with something that is so pure and so clear in its message: this is a matter of life and death. We will turn America around. We are changing the attitude of the American people by bringing them something beautiful. There is nothing beautiful about AIDS. It is a hideous disease. It does hideous things to people's bodies and minds. With The Quilt, we're able to touch people in a new way and open their hearts so that they no longer turn away from it, but rather understand the value of all of these lost lives.

Cleve Jones, executive director of The NAMES Project

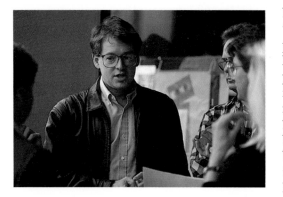

"Our community and our ideals will survive this epidemic," predicts Cleve Jones. "I may not be around to see it, but we will defeat AIDS."

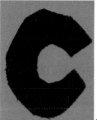leve Jones doesn't sew, and The Quilt was only a vague idea in his mind on February 20, 1987, when he went into his backyard with cans of spray paint, stencils and a white sheet to make a memorial for Marvin Feldman, Cleve's best friend of 14 years who had died of AIDS four months earlier. "I spent the whole afternoon thinking about Marvin," remembers Cleve. "I thought about why we were best friends and why I loved him so much. By the time I finished the piece, my grief had been replaced by a sense of resolution and completion."

Cleve felt particularly comforted when he thought of Marvin's memorial as a quilt. "There's promise in a quilt," says Cleve. "It's not a shroud or a tombstone. It's so important for people whose greatest enemy is despair. I really believe that the worst thing that could happen to us is to despair and to stop living and loving and fighting."

Cleve Jones knows what it's like to be paralyzed with despair. By 1984, almost all of his friends were sick or had died of AIDS. "It was so clear that I was right in the center of the circle of people that were going to be hit the hardest," says Cleve, who has lived in San Francisco's predominantly gay Castro district for 15 years. "I wasn't just losing friends, but also losing all the familiar faces of the neighborhood — the bus drivers, clerks and mailmen. To me, Castro Street is populated by ghosts. When I walk up 18th Street from Church Street to Eureka Street, a distance of eight blocks, just looking at all these houses and knowing the stories behind so many of the windows, makes me feel so old. To know that's where Shane died, that's where Alan died, that was Bobby's last house, that's where Gregory died, that's where Jimmy was diagnosed, that's the house Alex got kicked out of . . . "

By the time of Marvin's death in late 1986, the grief was overwhelming. "I began to believe that there was no hope," he says, "and that everyone I cared about was going to die from this disease. I lost my sense of humor, and I lost my ability to fight back."

His old spirit returned with the launching of The NAMES Project. "I had become numb," he recalls. "When somebody you know dies every day, what do you do? You try to stop feeling and stop remembering. But I don't want to stop remembering Marvin Feldman and all the other friends of mine that have gone. They shaped my life and I love them and I don't want to forget them. I had to find a way for me to hold on to those memories and everything I cherish about those people."

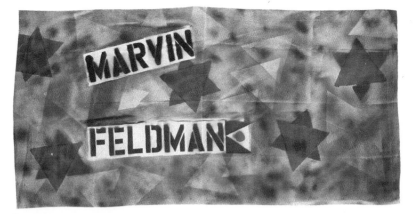

A Quaker background and years of political activism helped Cleve prepare for the Project. Cleve first became involved in gay rights politics during high school in his hometown of Phoenix, Arizona. Just after graduating in 1972, he "came out" to his sister and parents, both professors at Arizona State University, and moved to San Francisco. There, he became an 18-year-old rabble-rouser who helped organize gay pride midnight marches. Majoring in urban studies at San Francisco State University, Cleve served as a student intern for San Francisco Supervisor Harvey Milk. After Milk was murdered on November 27, 1978, Cleve helped organize the annual candlelight memorial marches down Market Street. Later, he served five years as a legislative consultant to Assemblyman Art Agnos, now San Francisco's mayor.

In April 1986, Cleve told a nationwide television audience that he was antibody positive to the AIDS virus on a "60 Minutes" program about San Francisco's response to the AIDS epidemic. He wanted, he says, to help demystify the disease. Four weeks later, two men, calling him "faggot," stabbed Cleve in the back as he neared his home in Sacramento. During his three months of recuperation, Cleve had time to think about organizing The Quilt, an idea that had long been floating around his head. Some friends thought the idea was morbid; others simply couldn't see how it would work. But after he joined forces with Mike Smith in May 1987, things started to click. They advertised The Quilt project across the country, and soon were being overwhelmed by the response. Hundreds of panels arrived to be sewn together with the painted cloth memorial Cleve had made for Marvin Feldman.

"The Quilt has helped me turn my back on cynicism," says Cleve. "I used to be constantly aware of the hurt, pain and evil people are capable of. The Quilt has helped me believe that in all of us there really is something that is very good. It's O.K. to get angry, it's O.K. to get impatient, it's O.K. to have fights, but it is important not to give up on people.

"It's such an evil thing that has happened," says Cleve, referring to the mothers and fathers who have to deal with ostracism from their neighbors while they are mourning their children. "To know that this project is reaching those people is just astonishing to me. The Quilt is pure good. That's what I love about it. People of goodwill, people with the heart capacity to get the message, just seem to blossom into it. So every part of the work ends up being so exciting."

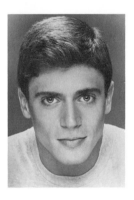

Cleve Jones dedicated The NAMES Project to 33-year-old actor Marvin Feldman, who died of AIDS in October 1986. He created the first panel for The Quilt in Marvin's honor.

Since July 1987, Cleve's life has been dedicated to his efforts to publicize The NAMES Project. In an endless round of interviews, he has sought to use The Quilt as a way to educate audiences across the country about AIDS, about grief, and about the cooperative spirit that created The Quilt. Something magical, he says, has come out of the process of sewing together a unique memorial. "You get this group of people in a room," he says, "and one is a telephone operator, another a word processor, a ballerina and a waiter, and you tell them that they've got to figure out a way to display ten tons of fabric. You leave them alone for an hour and when you come back they're laughing hysterically but they have a workable plan. It's just constantly marvelous.

"The Quilt is the best thing I have done in my life," Cleve says. A quote from Mother Teresa is pinned on the wall of his office cubicle. It reads: "There is a light in this world, a healing spirit more powerful than any darkness we may encounter. We sometimes lose sight of this force when there is suffering, too much pain. Then suddenly, the spirit will emerge through the lives of ordinary people who hear a call and answer in extraordinary ways."

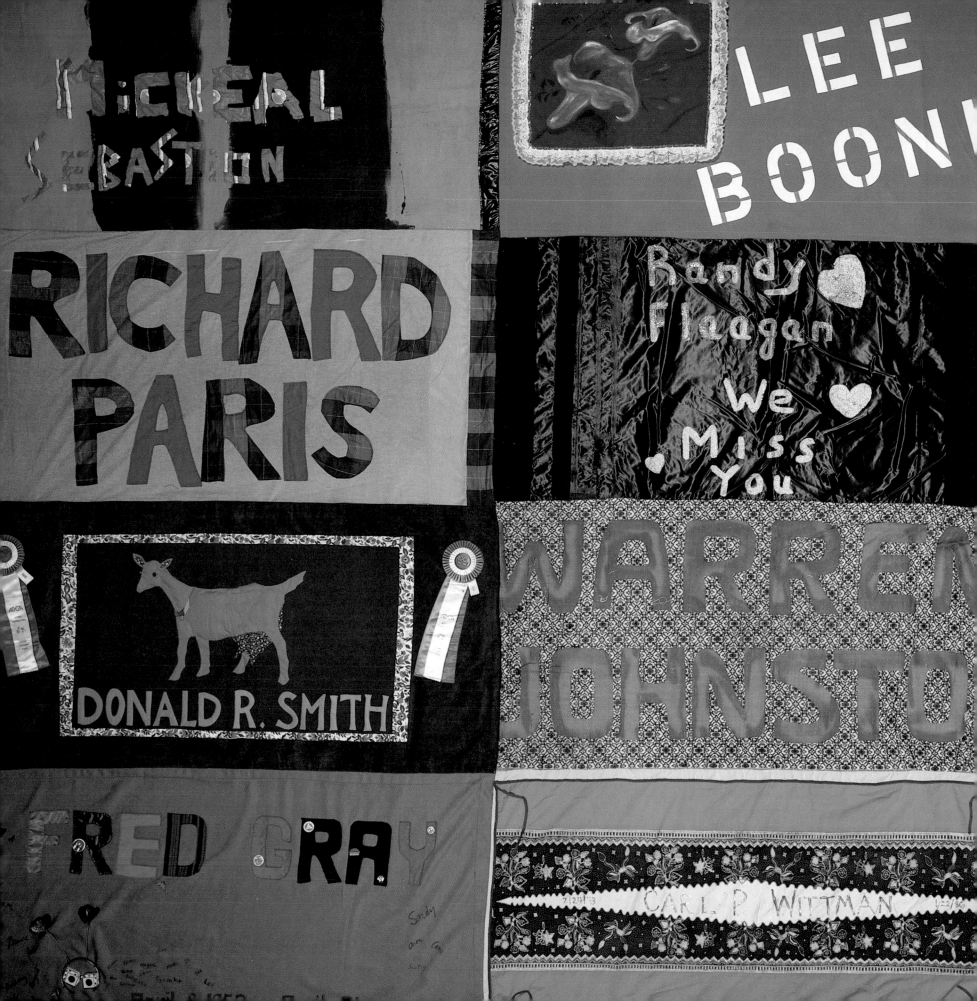

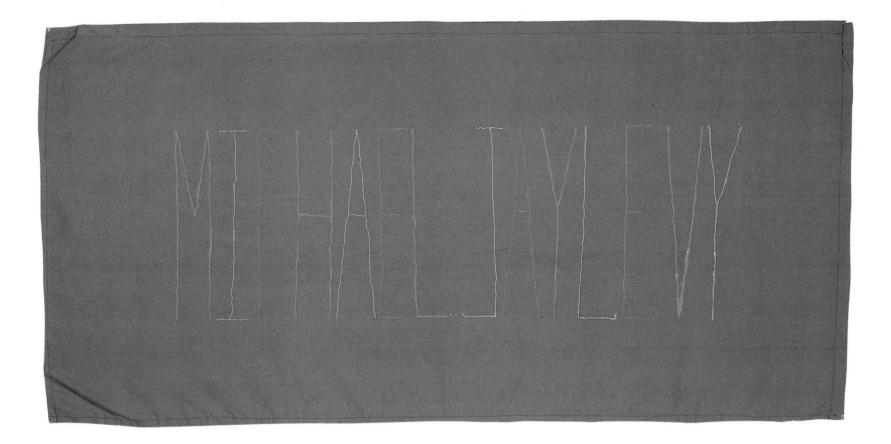

To honor Michael's memory
We sent this panel.

To give meaning to his death
We gain our strength from you.
To give hope to those afflicted,
Together, we shall fight the affliction.
To give strength to those left behind,
We look forward to better tomorrows.

He was our son.
He is all our brothers.
Our Michael is gone.
Try and save the others.

Michael's Parents, Pat and Mayer Levy
Chesterfield, Missouri
September 1987

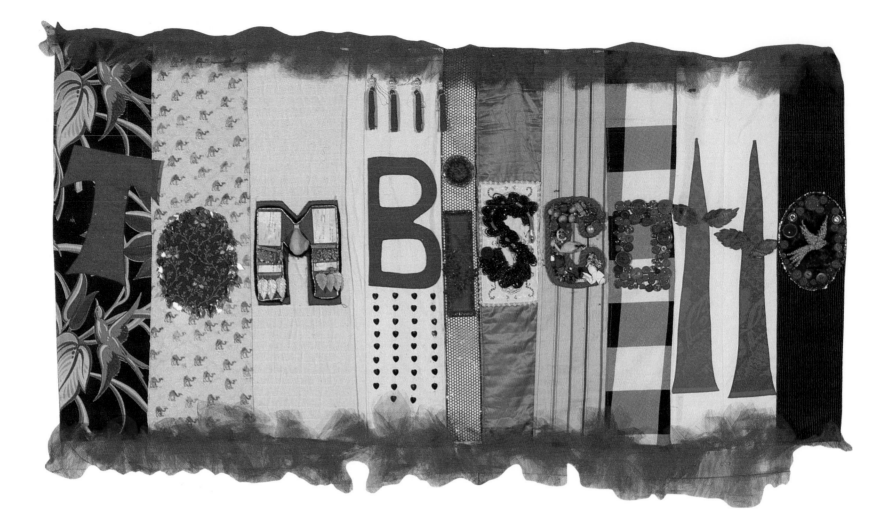

ourteen people worked on Tom Biscotto's panel with a different group designing each letter of his name. As the former stage manager of the Goodman Theater in Chicago — one of the country's top regional theaters — and cofounder of the Godzilla Rainbow acting troupe, Tom was a friend to many who had worked in the Chicago arts community. Jim Rinnert, Tom's lover of 13 years, orchestrated the efforts, in some cases contacting friends that Jim hadn't heard from since Tom's death in October 1984. The letters of Tom's name are laid out on a piece of the curtain that used to hang in Tom and Jim's house on Orchard Street in Chicago. The house was filled with plants, stuffed animals, live snakes and birds. Even Tom's enormous macaw, Gladys, contributed a feather to the panel. The Orchard Street house was, as one friend put it, "the haven for every lost artistic soul that passed through Chicago for over twenty years."

We don't think Tom needs to be memorialized in any way. He lives in each and every one of our hearts each and every day. He's been gone now for almost three years to the day and we think and speak of him no less than when he was with us in the flesh. Which should tell us something . . . he is still with us. And I'll tell you how we know . . . it was Tom that whispered in our ear that he thought the thing needed a little red tulle around the edges to finish it off.

And you know what? He's right!

Anne

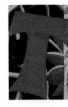 Jim Rinnert created the initial "T."

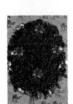 Lily, an actress in the Godzilla Rainbow troupe, hand-stamped the "O" with camels as a reminder of a trip she took to Morocco with Tom. On the trip, Tom kiddingly accepted a local merchant's offer of 4,000 camels in exchange for Lily.

 Kib, a friend from Toronto, chose birchbark and snakeweeds for the "M" to symbolize Tom's earthiness. According to friends, the nose is an exact replica of Tom's.

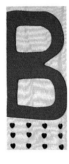 Tom's mother and sister Barb decorated the "B" in Los Angeles. After nursing him through the final months of his life, they set the sparkling hearts in lines as a symbol of their tears.

 Brent, a neighbor, dotted the "I" with a real pressed flower sealed in plastic, a stand-in for the indoor jungle that filled Tom's home.

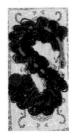 Anne, a onetime roommate of Jim and Tom's, included a snake in her design for the "S" to represent Rosie, the smaller of Tom's two boa constrictors. Anne remembers how the 15-foot boa lazed about on the kitchen counter, and she will never forget the time Rosie escaped and found refuge in the walls of the Orchard Street house. The background fabric, which Tom bought once for a costume, commemorates Tom's life in the theater. "The sequins are there," says Anne, "because if anyone loved glitz and truly appreciated its trashiness, it was Tom."

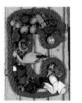 Greg Kooper designed the "C" in keeping with his and Tom's hippie phase in the 60s when they learned beading and macramé.

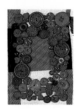 Charlotte, a neighbor, chose buttons for the "O" to recall Tom's ever-expanding collection of colorful buttons, beads, and trinkets that he picked up in his travels and then scattered all over the house.

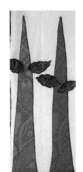 Jim, Richard, Virgie and Christina, friends now living together in Sawyer, Indiana, organized their own sewing bee to design the double "T."

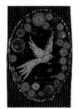 The final "O" was made by Deb and Gusto, tenants that lived upstairs from Tom.

In the panel's final phase, Jim, Anne and Lily gathered together the separate pieces created by Tom's far-flung friends and family. Late one night, while playing Tom's records, drinking, laughing a lot and crying a little, they sewed the pieces together and spelled out the name of their friend.

y the time real estate broker Paul Burdett was 28, he owned five apartment buildings and a commercial office building. He lived in a San Diego home that he personally designed. Paul was the inspiration and the organizer of the first 50-hour AIDS Vigil at his church. His parents chose this achievement for his panel.

Together, Paul's parents discussed what to write on the commemorative panel they made for their only son, eventually deciding on "Please — More Prayers. More Funding." Paul's father, Fred Burdett, made the panel in Paul's favorite colors. On peach fabric, his father stenciled Paul's name in gray. With silver paint, he outlined all the letters and traced a computerized blowup photograph of his son in order to create a halo effect. Paul's mother embroidered the red heart at the bottom and handwrote "Love Mom and Dad."

A week before he died, Paul Burdett wrote a letter to his family and friends.

Dear Mom, Dad, Sandi, Andy, my beloved Tim, and all my family and friends,

I just had to write this letter to tell you how much I love and care for you. I have seen you moving through the past few days in a daze, crying and grieving so much that I thought that your hearts and my heart would break.

I spent many hours on the last day of my physical existence wrestling with God and trying to understand His will for me. Then Christ came, knelt by my bedside and asked me softly to take His hand. I looked in His eyes and realized that I had seen them before, throughout all my life, in each of you.

I saw you fall asleep last night with the moonlight shining on your face and I longed to touch your brow and let you know that I am finally at peace.

Paul.

Our message to parents is to say Please don't turn your backs on your sons and daughters. Give them your love and support while you can. We miss our son so very much.

Mr. & Mrs. F. Burdett

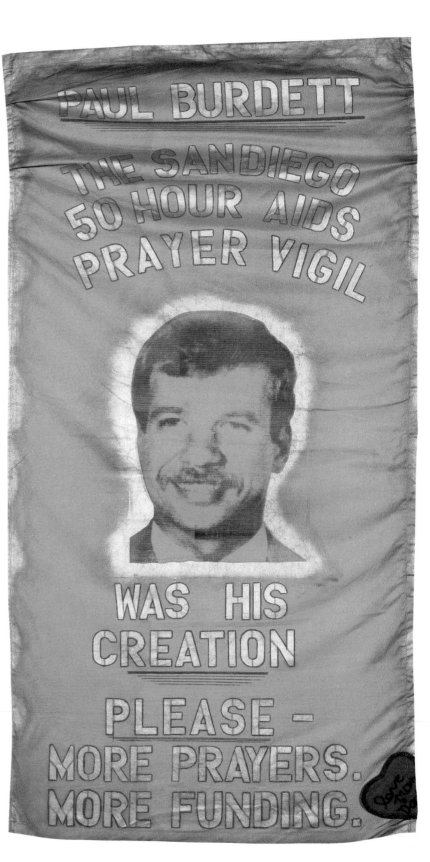

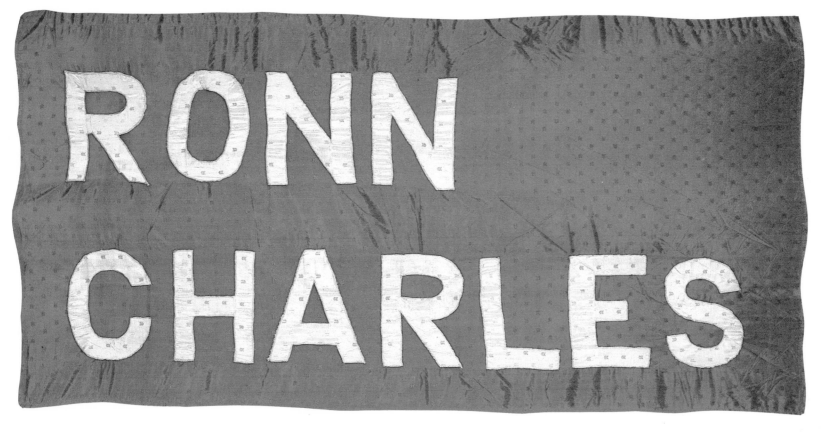

 onn Charles died in the arms of his sister Bobbe Rigler. When he had become too sick to care for himself, he moved from New York City to Mill Valley, California, to be with Bobbe, her husband and their two children. He wanted to spend his last months with family.

Friends and relatives visited constantly while Ronn was ill. They hugged him, kissed him, bathed him and fed him. After having so many people around while her brother was dying, Bobbe chose to make his memorial alone. "It was something I had to do for myself. I didn't want to include anyone else."

Bobbe stenciled Ronn's name in large silver-gray block letters onto a red silk fabric. "My brother was a real class act," she says. "So I wanted the panel to be real simple, just like him." As she stitched, she realized how glad she had been to fulfill her brother's last request — to die with respect and dignity in their home rather than in a hospital. After she sewed the last letter on, she cried. "I thought I was being really brave," she says. "But when I saw his name all laid out, I just broke down."

I shall always remember his final gift to me and my family — that he chose us to live his final days with, and our home to die in. He added love, understanding, compassion and humor to our lives. I shall miss him always.

Bobbe Rigler

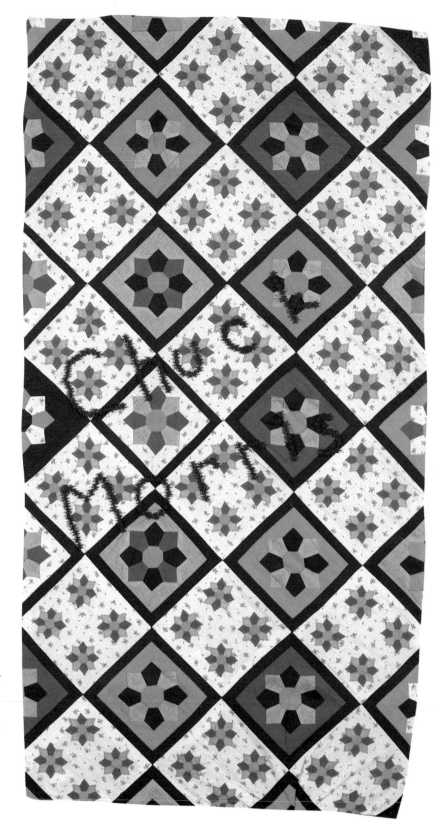

It is amazing — even eerie — that the unfinished quilt pattern was exactly the size of the panels you are seeking. It is somehow like Chuck knew unconsciously where the quilt would end up, long before The NAMES Project existed. All the handwork is his. He made his own panel.

Janet Lewallen
Denver, Colorado

26

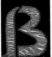y the time Charles Lee Morris was 40, he had worked as a foreign correspondent for CBS News, managed Gore Vidal's U.S. senatorial bid in 1972, and served on a myriad of civic councils, executive committees and mayoral commissions in San Francisco. But he is best known as the publisher of *The Sentinel*. He transformed this small newspaper serving San Francisco's gay community into a hard-news weekly in the vanguard of the gay press. *The Sentinel* was the first newspaper in the country to run a story on a rare form of pneumonia and cancer that had inexplicably afflicted a number of gay men.

Chuck was diagnosed with AIDS early in 1982, and by 1984 he chose to turn away from his fast-paced public life by moving to Denver to join his new lover, James Swope. As part of his quieter life-style in Colorado, Chuck learned how to sew. For two years, Chuck worked on a quilt, spending eight to ten hours a day quilting in the traditional style. He wondered what people from his San Francisco heyday would think if they could see him now, chatting up the ladies in sewing stores for pointers. Chuck did not complete the quilt, but when he died it was precisely three by six feet — the exact size required by the still-to-be-formed NAMES Project.

Chuck's lover, Jim didn't know what to do with the unfinished quilt. For the first month, he slept with it. Then he packed it away in a drawer, taking it with him when he moved to West Palm Beach, Florida. A year and a half after Chuck's death, Jim received a call from Jan, a close friend who wanted to know whether she could make a NAMES Project panel for Chuck. "I think that it is basically made," replied Jim. He mailed the quilt to Jan. She merely added a backing and spelled out Chuck's name in little red plastic flowers.

I met Chuck Morris several years after he had been diagnosed with AIDS. I don't remember how it all happened, but I remember being absolutely knocked over by this gangly guy who tipped the scales at 106 pounds. We were inseparable from the first. It was as if we had always been in love.

I was terrified to find myself in love with a man who had this creepy, deadly, contagious disease. I didn't know what was happening. All I knew was that being with him was where I wanted to be, that love was indeed all that it was cracked up to be. I knew Chuck wasn't healthy, but I couldn't think of him as sick. Nothing was wrong with his mind, nothing wrong with his spirit.

No one can ever tell if a relationship is going to work, and everything was stacked up against us. We lived a thousand miles apart. For many hours, with many people, I talked about committing myself to a dying man, and ended inviting Chuck to move in with me.

He immediately brought domesticity to my life. Coming home after dark to see the lights already on was a second gift. My apartment became our home. We were so happy together! We spent evenings sitting quietly together, working on projects. He decided to make me a quilt — this quilt. He amazed himself, stitching as intently as he used to editorialize, but it never got finished.

When Chuck died, accolades came in from all over. He was credited with elevating the professionalism of the gay press, and of being a leader in the community. His death made front page news in Denver, and friends sent me articles clipped from papers across the country. Although I knew about those things, and was proud of Chuck for them, they weren't what was important to me.

He made me confront my values, my motives, and my desires. As my love for him grew, so did my love for myself.

He was 42 years old when he died. He died at home, broken in body but with a legacy of accomplishments far beyond his too few years. We were together two years and two days.

James Swope

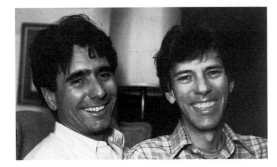

Chuck Morris (right) with Jim Swope.

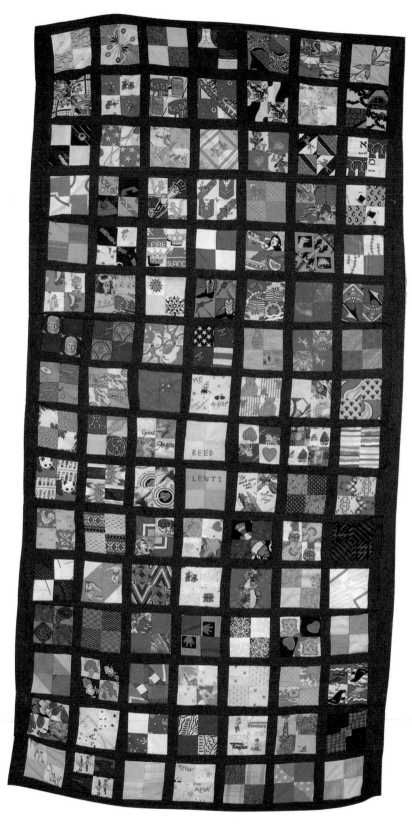

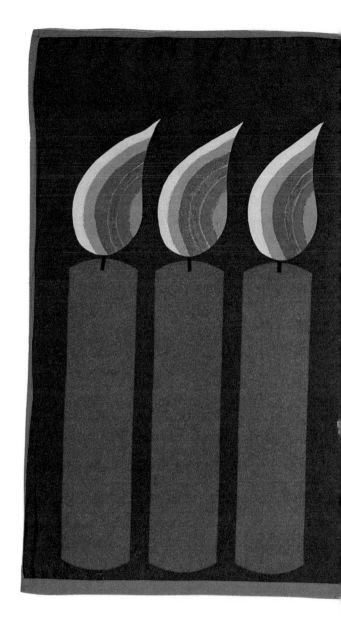

Alan Isaksen placed his lover's name, Reed Lenti, in the center of his quilt surrounded by fabric from friends and places they had shared over their 11 years together, including napkins from favorite restaurants, fabric picked up on trips to Greece and Egypt, pieces of their own clothes, and remnants from friends. Alan has collected fabric for 15 years, diligently documenting the name of the person or the place that it came from.

JOHN BOOTH

"To 12 men I expected to grow old with," Lance Hecox wrote on the back of this memorial. "Nine who have passed on and three who will join them soon." Since making the panel, two of the remaining candles have been extinguished. The first candle is for Jim Howell, the fourteenth official AIDS patient in the U.S., and now, seven years later, 35-year-old Lance is taking care of Robert, the last of this group of friends.

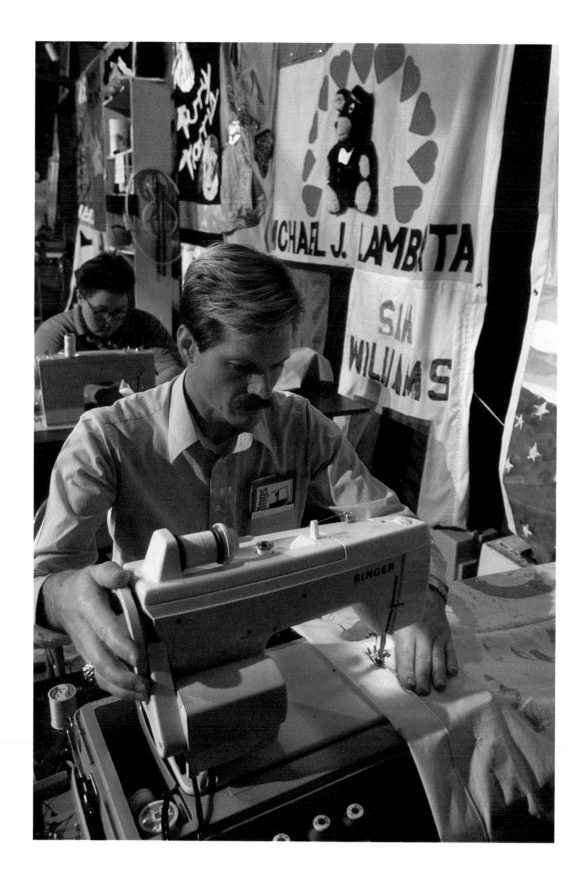

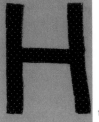uddled over a sewing machine, four of Ron Carey's close friends stitch his tasseled cowboy shirt, a drawing, and his name in huge letters on a cloth panel. At a nearby table, an 11-year-old boy draws a rainbow over the Golden Gate bridge, and with a thick red felt marker he carefully traces the name of his father's lover who died of AIDS two years ago. A woman weeps as she pastes felt letters and glitter on floral fabric, spelling out the name of her brother. Ron Cordova, technical director of The NAMES Project, drops his pinking shears and comforts her. This is a very special sewing circle: tears flow constantly in The NAMES Project workshop, a place where people create quilts in memory of a loved one they have lost to AIDS.

The shelves along the back wall of the workshop overflow with donated cloth, fur, feathers and sequins. "When Donghia Fabrics donated boxes of beautiful material, it was like opening a treasure chest," Scott Lago, the workshop's production manager, says over the chatter, the whir of sewing machines and Bronski Beat blaring from the tape deck.

At a three-by-six-foot table, two men can't decide what to do on their friend's quilt panel: should they use the gold lamé and shocking pink feather boa for his more flamboyant side, or the flannel and teddy bears for his warm, snugly nature?

Jim Poche, who has AIDS, is working on his fourth panel. "Being here is very difficult," says Jim. "I'm faced with my own mortality. You do your best to pretend you're not sick, but when you're in a room with the names of your friends, you wonder how much longer you'll have the strength to continue the battle." Jim is cheered up by little Ruby Cymrot, going on three, who bounces from sewing machine to sewing machine. She squeals with delight as Cleve Jones chases her in and out of the bolts of fabric, threatening to pop the purple balloon attached to her red corduroy overalls. Ruby, her curly mop of hair done up with ribbons and a sprinkling of sequins, has come in with her mother and Dafna Wu, her mother's lover, to make a panel for Matsuko Gaffney. Barbara and Dafna don't know anyone personally who has died of AIDS, but checked into the Project to see if anybody wanted help making panels. "It was important to me that Matsuko be incorporated in the quilt," says Dafna of the Asian woman who was infected with the virus from a blood transfusion. "This is not only a gay, white man's disease."

High school sophomore Rebecca Sweet is pasting feathers and sequins on a panel for her friend Carlos. Rebecca, a full-time summer volunteer who hems materials and welcomes visitors,

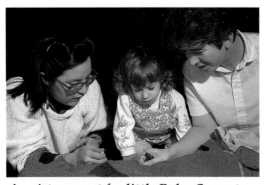

A quiet moment for little Ruby Cymrot as she watches her mother (right) and quilter Dafna Wu work on a panel together.

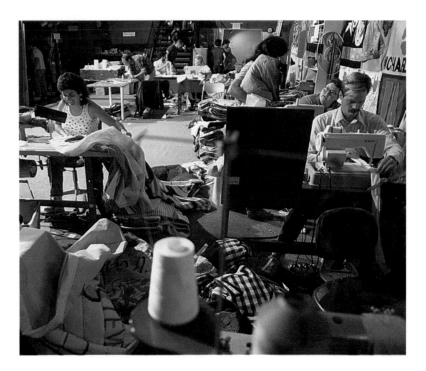

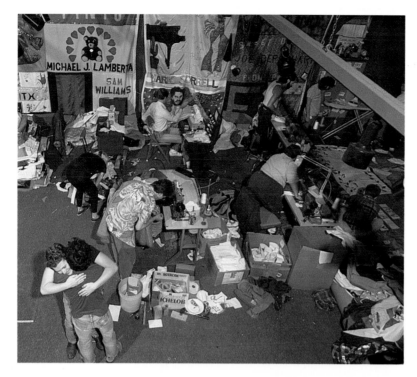

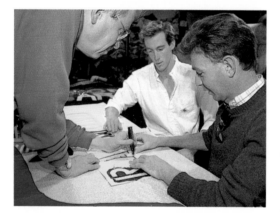

has made seven panels. Willi "Jack" Heard answers the phone at the information desk. Willi, a 12-year-old who says that he likes to act like an adult, doesn't tell his schoolmates where he spends his afternoons. "It's personal," he says. "I'm just trying to help out. I'd be embarrassed that kids would tease me." Willi is cutting out a stencil for the quilt panel he is making for Kail, a friend of his mother's. "I love art," he says, "and I can relate to the people here, especially Cleve. He jokes around a lot. He's very warm. He's cool. He's gnarly."

A mother and her son bring in a panel the family have made for Robert Lee Campbell, Jr. "It's so difficult giving the panel up," she says in tears. A volunteer hangs it from the balcony railing next to the sequined panel for Rock Hudson. A group of tourists linger around the windows, and a few venture in, curious about this storefront full of names, color and excitement. "This is the most eloquent expression of love," remarks a visitor from Ohio.

The offices on a second-floor balcony overlook the buzzing work area below. Cleve Jones is talking to a reporter. Mike Smith, general manager of The NAMES Project, is juggling telephone calls. Mike Smith holds The NAMES Project together, charging Project bills to his personal credit cards. On one line he is arranging for permits with Park Service officials in Washington for the inaugural display of The Quilt, on another he discusses printing costs for a program, and on a third line he explains the Project's urgency to a possible funding source. Crumpled under his desk is the panel Mike started working on three months ago for Jeff, a Stanford Business School classmate who died of AIDS during second-year finals.

Word processor Dan Carmell, entering information about the panels into a computer, is sobbing. "I can't help getting emotional," says the 28-year-old inventory coordinator.

Danny Sauro, the media director, leans over the mezzanine banister, watching the people making quilt panels below. Danny left his job as a market researcher for CBS in New York in May 1986, to be with his lover, Garth, a personnel psychologist for the army. Seven months later Garth was diagnosed with AIDS. "The only solid, safe thing in my life," says Dan, "is that I had Garth — and then he was diagnosed." After Danny saw Cleve's "Wish List" in the window of the workshop, he emptied his desk and returned with a box of pencils, pens and paper clips. In his capacity as media coordinator for The NAMES Project, Danny found a place to do something meaningful.

Ron Cordova immediately put volunteer Steve Newberger to work pinning and hemming. Only two days earlier, Steve had handed in his panel for Baird Underhill unhemmed because he didn't know how to use a sewing machine. He raises his hand for help threading his machine. Full-time volunteer Cindy McMullin with two-toned hair, black leggings, a brooch crafted from a spool of mauve thread and a jangling bracelet of bobbins comes over to help Steve.

Eve M. slips in quietly, takes her place behind a machine and begins piecing panels together. Her boyfriend died of AIDS two weeks earlier. Soon she is laughing and singing a rendition of "There's No Business Like Sew Business" with Scott and Cindy. Eve cared for her boyfriend Roger for two years. The day after he died, Roger's family claimed his apartment and possessions. They wanted no contact with Eve, so she left quickly, with no farewell ceremony to him and no mementos. She lived in a daze until a friend brought her to The NAMES Project workshop. "I came in moping and sad," she says. "But then I walked into this busy-bee place, and in a couple of days, it became my whole life. It's all I live for. To come here, to touch the panels . . . to feel them. Even though I'm not a good seamstress, I was needed and that felt good."

Jack Caster returns from the post office with a dozen parcels. Three panels were packaged together with a note attached asking that they be sewn side by side. The volunteers clear the center of the work space, and Ron begins to arrange eight panels to form a 12-by-12-foot square.

A staff meeting is called at 8 P.M. Forty volunteers pull chairs and beanbag pillows into a circle. Mike Smith lays out his panel for Jeff. This is the only opportunity he has to work on it. Sorting through the colors in his box of fabric scraps, Mike opens the meeting with a financial report. Scott, with an embroidery frame propped on his knee, is appliquéing a heart onto a commissioned panel. Debra Resnik, a 35-year-old full-time volunteer, doesn't leave her sewing machine. "I keep the panels face-down," says Debra, who loves to sew. "If I look at the names, I get too involved and I'd never get anything done." Ron announces excitedly that Henry Calvin Fabrics has donated 2,000 yards of white fabric for the walkways that will run between the quilt squares. "We are here to turn the country around," Cleve tells the volunteers. "We're going to bring the message of The Quilt to the American people. We're going to be in the history books and the art books. The level of hysteria — the hate, the mistrust, the fear — around AIDS has dropped way down. Each one of you can take some real credit for moving Americans toward greater compassion for people with AIDS."

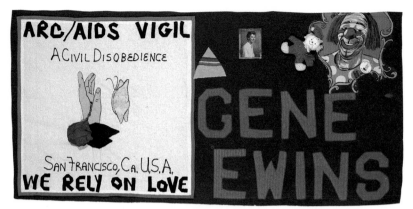

From the moment Terry Blankenship's ex-husband died in the summer of 1985, she knew that she wanted to help other people with AIDS. Terry moved from Winchester, Kentucky, to San Francisco, where she lived in a tent at the ARC/AIDS Vigil for five months. She wanted to memorialize two men who camped out with her at the Vigil, but since there were no lights or sewing machines at the camp site, Terry came into the workshop. "This is a love story," says Terry, looking at the clusters of people sewing around her. "This is also a story about fear, sorrow . . . and a medical emergency. There are an awful lot of unseen people that are affected by this. Sooner or later it will touch each one of us. We're all part of one big family — we're the folks next door."

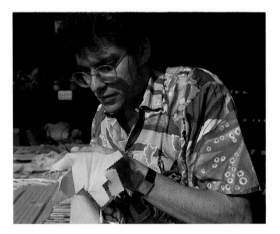

Scott Lago, The NAMES Project authority on sewing techniques and quilt trivia, diligently creates cutouts with his pinking shears.

33

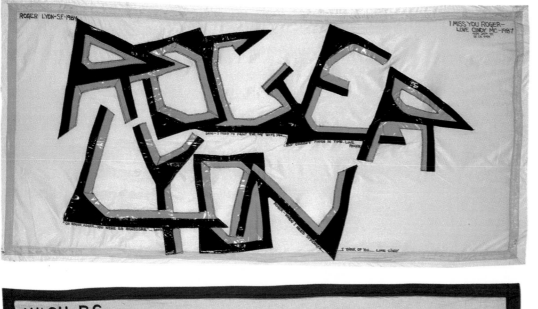

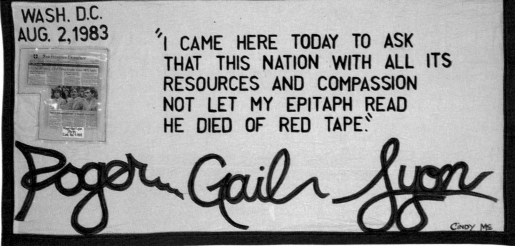

While Roger Lyon, a well-known AIDS activist, was ill with AIDS, he was asked to speak to a fifth-grade class at a San Francisco Catholic school. The children, in turn, made him get-well cards.

"Dear Roger," one student wrote. "I think you will get out of this tuff spot."

"Dear Roger," wrote another. "You better get well soon, else you owe me $5.00 for my time and effort."

Cindy McMullin met Roger through her friend David, who was Roger's lover. Almost three years after Roger's death in 1984, Cindy became one of the first sewing volunteers at The NAMES Project. By day she sold men's cologne at Macy's and at night she sewed quilt panels. "Usually when I got out of work I'd be really wiped out, but when I came to The NAMES Project I didn't want to leave," she says. "I'm so pleased, so honored when people ask me to help them with their panels — I know how personal it is." After The Quilt's inaugural display in Washington, Cindy gave up her day job to work full-time at The NAMES Project.

"I never do stuff like this. I've never volunteered before," she confesses. "But now I'm turning into the kind of person I used to hate. I'm always wearing my NAMES Project pin and my badges, and approaching people on the street with posters and pamphlets."

So far, Cindy has made seven panels. She made three of them in honor of Roger Lyon. Carefully she traced the get-well cards from the fifth-graders onto one panel. Roger never saw the cards. They arrived the day after he died.

34

Roger,

The day I met you, my best friend of ten years told me he had fallen madly in love with you and that you would be living together. Oh yes, and that you had AIDS.

Oh Roger — please forgive me for the ten minutes that it took me to stop hating you. I didn't know you and all I could feel was anger and then panic that David might become ill. And I had loved him for so long and I didn't know you at all!

Memories of you are not ones most people share. Wheelchairs, hospital waiting rooms, watching you fall, trying to help you up without you being mad that someone had to help you, watching you sleep, and (the most fun!) talking about all of David's faults and nasty habits while lying in bed.

Few memories, true . . . but what I have is all stored very tenderly in my heart.

Roger, I have learned one thing in my life. Don't get to know someone and become friends after they die. I never got the chance to run and play with you or to watch you have the time to be happy.

You have given me one thing — a determination to be the kind of person you would admire. One who touches, wants to be touched and cares. Your respect is my ultimate goal.

Love you so, Cindy

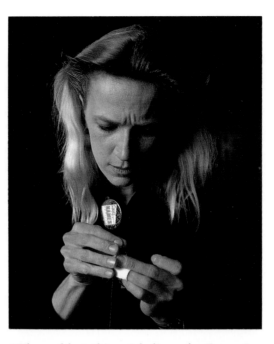

"The saddest thing, I believe, for Roger Lyon," says Cindy McMullin, "was how unfair it was to have to die without knowing how it — AIDS — is all going to end."

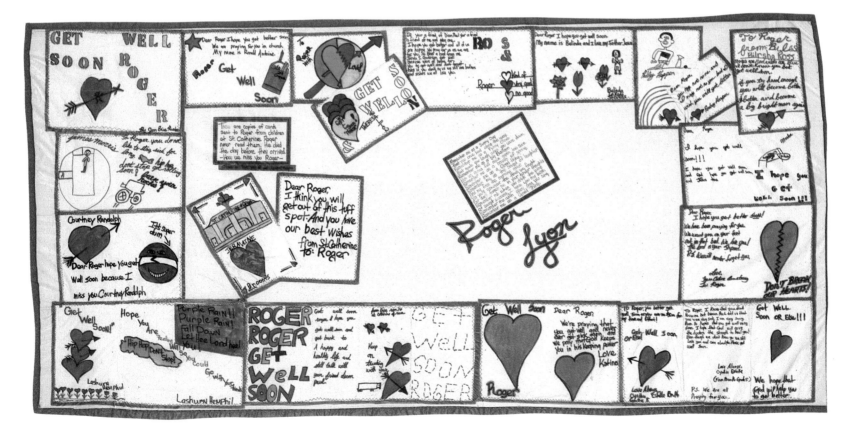

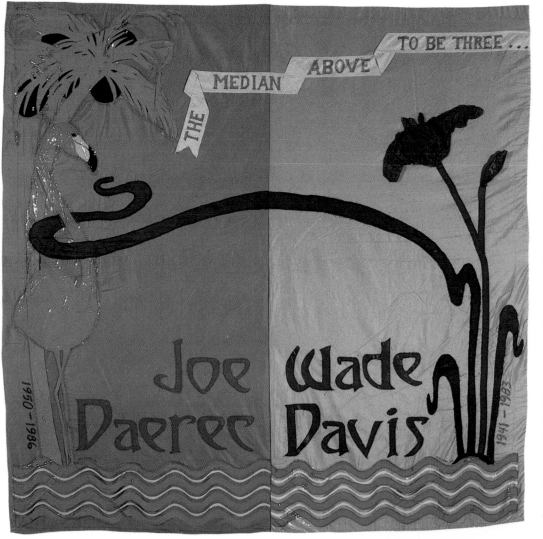

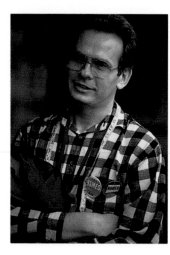

J ack Caster had two lifetime partners, Wade Davis and Joe Daerec. Eleven years ago, they moved from Detroit to San Francisco together, where they bought a house on Golden Gate Park and opened an art nouveau furniture business. Now Jack is alone. In 1983, after living with Jack for 17 years, Wade died of AIDS. Joe died three years later. "My grief was so intense that I was ready to die," says Jack, 44. "My pain was very personal. My friends' deaths felt different — they were so much more than two AIDS statistics."

Now a full-time volunteer at The NAMES Project workshop, Jack decorated Wade and Joe's panels with a pink flamingo and plastic waves cut out of their shower curtain. An art nouveau trim of whiplash iris leaves holds the two panels together. "I never knew any of these people four months ago," Jack says, looking around the bustling sewing room. "Now I know 230 new people, and so many are my very close friends. I feel connected. Everyone I meet here has suffered the same loss that I have. We cry together, but there is also constant laughter. For the first time since Wade got sick almost six years ago, I'm having fun."

Jack, who is coordinator of The Quilt's national tour, often finds himself comforting the parents who have lost their children to AIDS. "My own mother is supportive," says Jack, who is feeling well but is nevertheless anxious about his probable risk, "but when I talked with her about AIDS and The Quilt, it was like we were talking in the third person. I told her that we were going on tour to reach the families — the mothers. I didn't say that it was for her as well. Yet I got the feeling she knew . . . it was a strange feeling."

"The NAMES Project saved my life," says full-time volunteer Jack Caster.

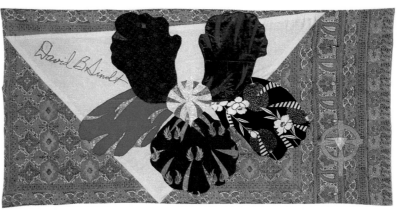

Andrew Weber, a freshman at Macalester College in St. Paul, Minnesota, designed this panel for his uncle David with help from his mother and an artist friend Lone Jensen. David Sindt was an avid iris grower. Andrew chose a significant fabric for each petal to symbolize a member of his family: the blue Indonesian batik is for David; the red satin is for his brother Dan; the purple satin is for his mother Claire, David's sister; the Japanese print is for his father; and the black and copper-colored print is from the cummerbund and bow tie Andrew wore to his high school senior prom.

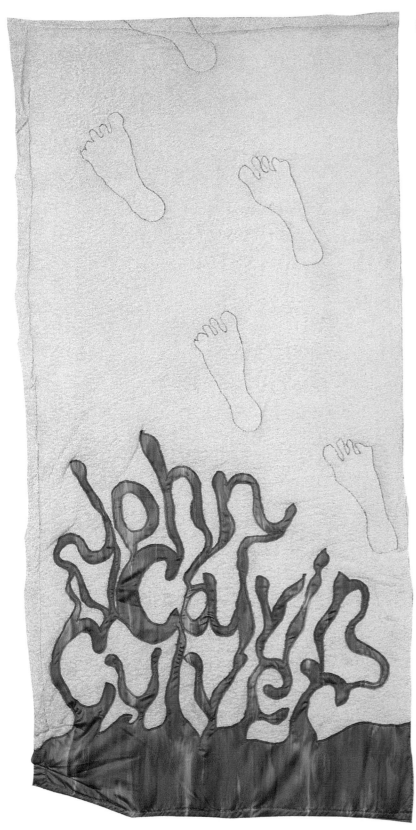

In rainbow-patterned taffeta on sand-colored terry cloth, John Wilson appliquéd the name of erotic film star John Calvin Culver, also known as Casey Donovan, to echo the title of one of his films made in the early 70s, Boys in the Sand. "He portrayed a positive sexy image," says Wilson, "at a time when it was dangerous to do so."

37

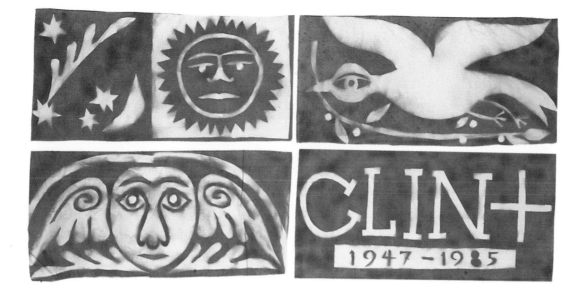

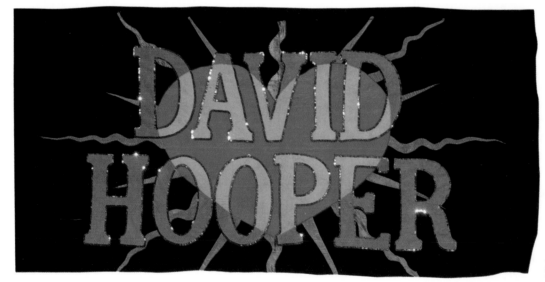

Bill Summers, a transportation orderly at Kaiser Hospital, San Francisco, organized a sewing bee of colleagues to honor 18 hospital employees who had died of AIDS. "In our profession, we learn to deal with illness and death by blocking out our personal feelings," says Bill. "But we were devastated when we realized how many of our fellow employees had died. One day they were working beside us, and they became our patients the next. We suffered silently as we lost each one." Nurse Susan Hansen assembled the panels (right) for eight Kaiser nurses she worked with.

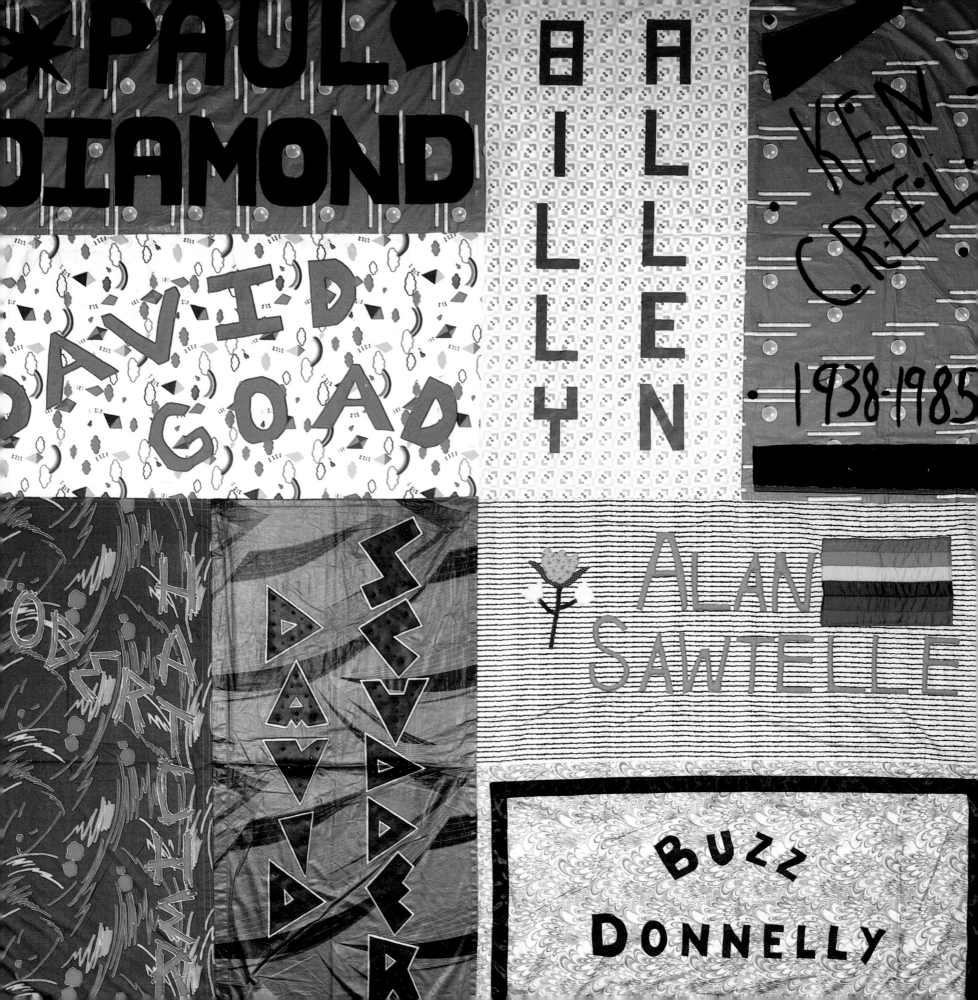

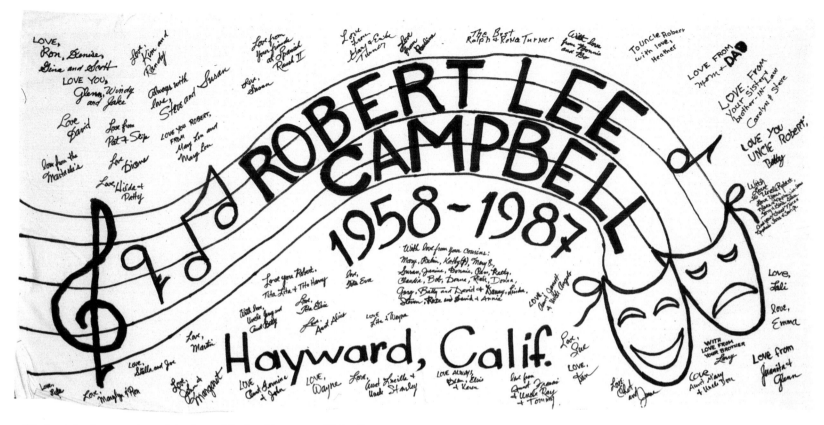

"Robert had a great need to have his family around him," says his brother Larry. "Everyone signed the panel because it was the last opportunity for the whole family to be with him. While our expressions of love are in the panel, they can't overshadow Robert himself."

When Robert's father tried to sign the panel, he was so distraught that he could barely form the letters needed to write "Dad."

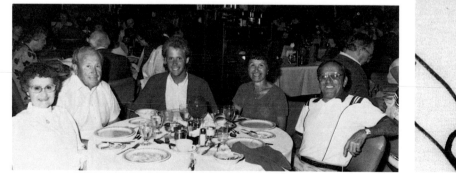

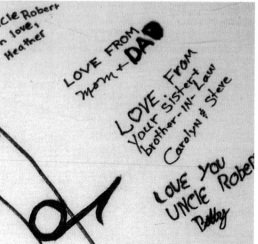

The Campbells have always been a very close-knit family. Robert Lee Campbell's grandfather, great-uncles and great-aunts lived on the same street in San Leandro, California. "Always the main thing was family," says Robert's older brother Larry. "We are family. We are one."

Robert's family never doubted that Robert was on his way to becoming a celebrity. As a little boy, he would spend hours in front of the television watching old MGM musicals, dreaming of show business. He could recite every episode of "I Love Lucy." At 13, he was the youngest person in the industry at that time to have his own television show. He started off as a weatherman, then became a game show announcer, and later landed a job as a talk show host. Still in high school, he interviewed Charlton Heston, Alfred Hitchcock, Henry Fonda, Edward Kennedy and Ava Gardner, among others. By the time he was 23, he was singing, dancing and acting in Hollywood clubs.

Robert wrote scripts for CBS's "Guiding Light" and spent two years as a cruise ship entertainer. He was rehearsing a cabaret act in New York when he collapsed with pneumonia. He flew back to his parents' home in Hayward, California, and on May 13, 1987, at Robert's request, the entire family gathered in his hospital room.

Twenty people, including his sisters' children, crowded in the small room. Robert lay in a fetal position wearing an oxygen mask and shivering while the doctor told those gathered that Robert would never recover. The doctor carefully explained his diagnosis — Robert didn't want anyone to have secondhand information.

Once the family knew that he had AIDS, Robert wanted to tell them that he was gay. But he put it off another two months. The Campbells are an old-world family. When Robert finally told them that he was gay, his parents were shaken. "It's a very hard thing for them," says Larry, now a high school teacher in San Jose. "At first when Robert was open about it, they were open about it. Then, too many of their friends made derogatory remarks. Now they don't even say that he died of AIDS, they say that he died of pneumonia."

The last time Robert went to the hospital he could no longer walk. His 73-year-old father, a retired roofing contractor, carried Robert to the car. "Please not yet," begged Robert, "don't take me to the hospital. I know that I am not coming back home again."

Once in the hospital, an anxious and tense Robert turned to his big brother. Larry had survived two near-death experiences of his own while being operated on for blood clots in his lungs. Now Robert wanted Larry to tell him exactly what it had been like.

"There's going to be so much open emotion around you and it's going to be scary. You're going to want to hold on," Larry warned.

"If I'm given the choice," answered Robert, "the way you were, I'll have to turn it down. I can't take any more of this pain. Please promise me that when it's time to go, you will be honest and let me know."

After their talk, a calmness came over Robert. Two days later he could no longer speak. He just kept staring at Larry. No matter where Larry moved, his eyes followed. His mother realized that the moment had come to leave Robert and Larry alone.

"Robert, I won't lie to you," Larry said quietly. "I know that you're scared and tired, but it's time now."

The two brothers held hands and went through benediction and prayers and then Larry said, "I can only walk so far with you and then you will have to walk over to the other side alone. Do you understand what I am saying?" Robert squeezed Larry's hand and tears trickled down his face. As he watched his brother die, Larry continued to speak. "Robert," he whispered, "I know you're on the other side. Soon you'll no longer hear me. I love you. We all do. The pain will stop. It's safe now."

Following Robert's death, the Campbell family shared its closeness and sadness in a typically unified way: parents, siblings, aunts, uncles, cousins, nieces and nephews all joined Robert's friends in signing a quilt panel in his memory. Larry flew to New York and Hollywood to gather signatures. "I couldn't even get to everyone who wanted to sign it," he recalls. "My parents are still getting letters and cards from all over the world on a weekly basis from people who are just finding out." So many friends and relatives attended Robert's funeral that the service had to be held in two chapels with people packed in the lobby and spilling outside. "He knew that he was loved," Larry said at the ceremony, "and this was important for him."

Larry and his mother traveled together to San Francisco to deliver the memorial banner they made for Robert. As they handed it to a NAMES Project volunteer, his mother cried out, "Reagan likes to hide his head in the sand. His problem is here — not sending off missiles. What will make him understand?"

"It was hard to fold up the panel," says Larry. "It was like putting my brother away. Everything was cut so short for him. He was only 29 years old. There was so much that he was in the process of doing, and everything was just about to work out."

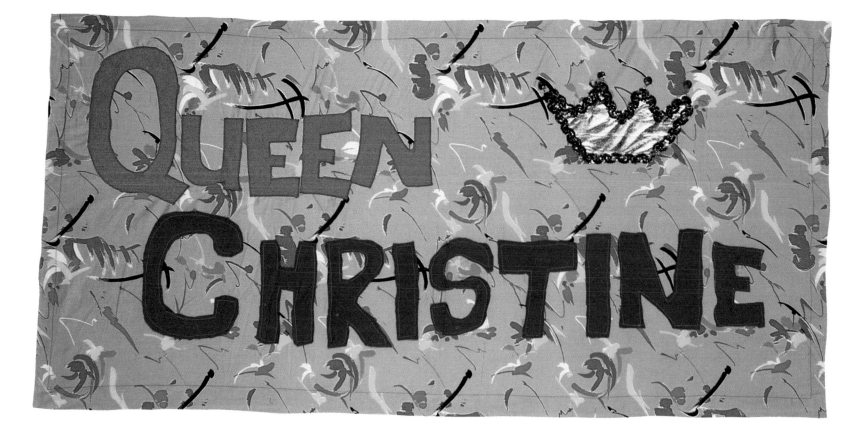

To be able to express my feelings in memory of a beautiful black woman who touched my heart with laughter is very special.

Christine Williams helped me understand that life isn't fair but that being honest with yourself and others can make a difference. God Bless you, Christine. You have helped me grow and want to survive.

Craig Pierce
San Francisco Hospice Nurse

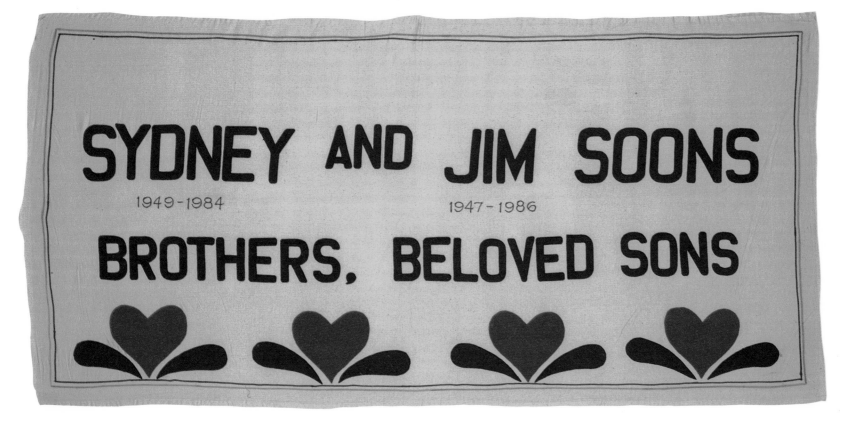

SYDNEY AND JIM SOONS
1949-1984   1947-1986
BROTHERS, BELOVED SONS

uring the summer of 1984 Sydney Soons, a hotel manager in Key West, Florida, phoned his 65-year-old mother, Judy. He wanted to come home for a visit. He warned his mother that he looked awful, yet she was still shocked when he arrived. She rushed him to a doctor, who predicted that he would be dead within a year. Sydney died in a hospital in Princeton, New Jersey, three months later.

The following summer, Jim, Judy's eldest son, came from Los Angeles to stay at the Soons' vacation home in Vermont. Despite the hot days, Jim wore long sleeves, trying to hide his lesions from his mother. Eventually Jim told her that he, too, had AIDS. They hugged, and Judy remembers him saying, "Mom, I feel so good that you know, and that I don't have to hide anything from you."

"We were sure that Jimmy would be the one to beat this awful thing, " Judy says wistfully. "Everything was an adventure and he had a great zest for life."

When Jim died in June 1986, Judy wrote to everyone on his Christmas list, as he instructed, and they all responded. Judy visits Jim and Sydney, buried next to each other in Princeton, with her remaining four children. Her daughter and one son are married. "I worry deeply about my other two," Judy says of her remaining gay sons. She also worries and shares mutual support with friends of Jim and Sydney who have called to say that they are sick. "Now I have so many gay friends," she says. "They stop by and hug me when I need to be hugged."

I do hope it's acceptable for me to put the names of both my sons on a single panel. Sydney and Jim would have approved because they were close friends. They are together in a lovely quiet place here in Princeton. I visit them often, tend their flowers, and find solace in the fact that their suffering is over and they are at peace.

Sydney was brightly intelligent with a wonderfully quick, whimsical sense of humor. Jim, with his flaming orange hair, was strong and energetic, exploding with adventurous spirit and a great zest for life.

I totally accepted the fact of their homosexuality. Unfortunately, the same cannot be said for their father, who is now my ex-husband.

Pray for all of us. I have two more gay sons. I live in fear.

Thank you,
Judy Soons

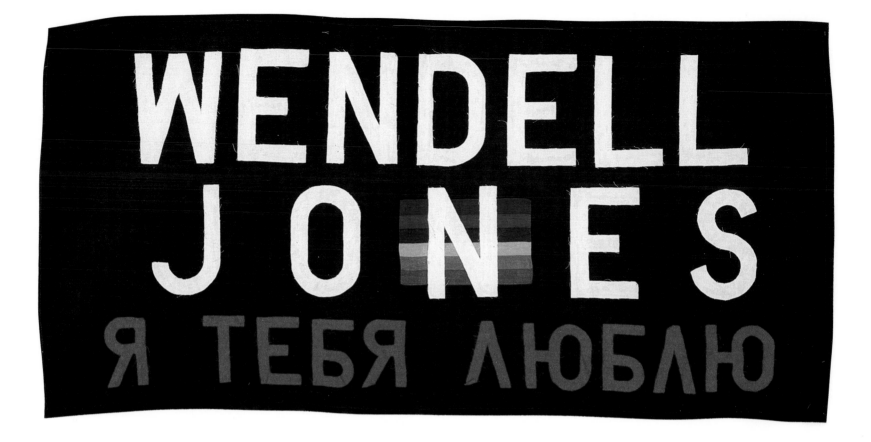

My Dearest Wendell,

I finished the panel dedicated to you for the AIDS quilt yesterday evening. It's not too fancy, but then again, you were always the more artistic half of our relationship. I spent a lot of time on it. I hope you like it and trust you don't mind me doing this.

Maybe I should describe it for you. It has a black background. I know, I know . . . how bleak! But your name is in huge white letters that you can see a mile away. I thought the black and white could symbolize our interracialness. There's a rainbow flag in the middle. Yes, it's the same one you gave me the year I marched with the Hayward float in the parade. I put something in red letters at the bottom in Russian. I wrote the phrase I taught you — I love you.

The panel will go to Washington, D.C., along with, I've been told, over 1,000 others. Remember how we both wanted to visit D.C. together? Well, it looks like, through the panel, you're getting the chance to see D.C. before me.

I guess I should close now. I hope you are O.K. You know, I see you when I look at the stars. Thank you for sharing three and a half miraculous years with me. I shall always, always love you, Wendell . . . my lover, my best friend.

Douglas Neil Payton, II

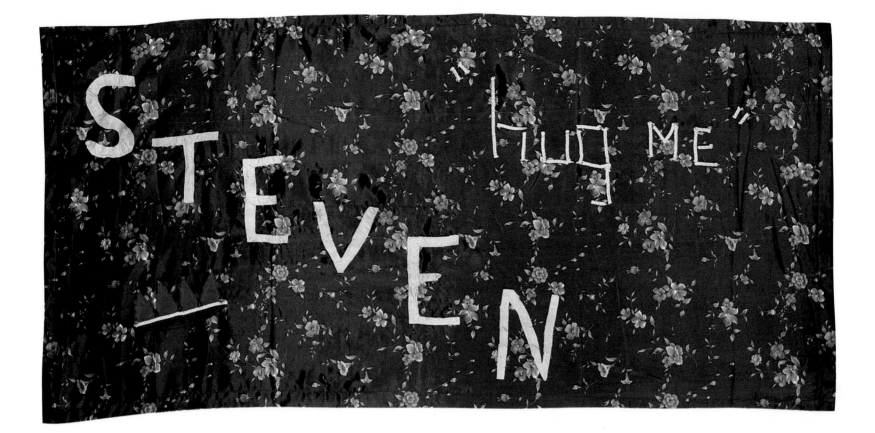

Steven had AIDS when I met him in 1981. We were all frightened about his sickness. He had been deserted by his lover and family. He was a very lonely man. We knew only that body fluids probably spread the virus but we didn't know what fluids. Steven had his silverware, plates and glasses separate, and he'd clean after himself. So much fear and ignorance then.

Once, he and I were dancing and when a slow song began to play, he begged for me to hold him and dance with him. To hug him. He was drenched in sweat, and he saw the fear in my face at coming in such close contact with him. It's 1987 now and I know that holding an AIDS victim is not going to give me the virus.

Vicki Hudson

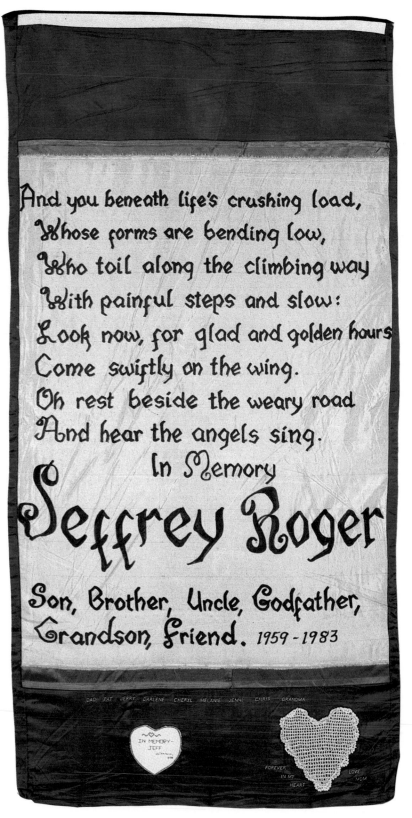

And you beneath life's crushing load,
Whose forms are bending low,
Who toil along the climbing way
With painful steps and slow:
Look now, for glad and golden hours
Come swiftly on the wing.
Oh rest beside the weary road
And hear the angels sing.
In Memory
Jeffrey Roger
Son, Brother, Uncle, Godfather,
Grandson, Friend. 1959-1983

DAD PAT JERRY CARLENE CHERYL MELANIE JENNI CHRIS GRANDMA

IN MEMORY — JEFF

FOREVER IN MY HEART   LOVE MOM

I had four sisters and I always wanted a brother. Jeff was born when I was 18 years old. I remember my Dad calling in tears from the hospital telling me that finally they had another son. Then I had to call him 23 years later to tell him that Jeff had died.

Jeff's brother, Jerry

hile in high school, Jeffrey Roger wrote letters constantly to his pen pal, Christopher, in Kansas. In 1978, he flew out to visit Chris for graduation, and they were soon in love. At 18, Jeff moved away from his family home in Milwaukee to live with Chris. Each December, the pair returned to Wisconsin to share a big family Christmas with Jeff's parents and five brothers and sisters.

In 1983, Jeff, 23, celebrated his last Christmas. He hadn't been feeling well since an accident he had at work a few years earlier. Operating machinery at Hallmark Greetings, Jeff had seriously mangled his left hand, an injury requiring repeated surgeries and skin grafts. Jeff's family believes he was infected with the AIDS virus by a contaminated blood transfusion.

Jeff's panel derived from one of the family's shared Decembers. In 1983, Jeff and Chris attended a Christmas Eve service in Milwaukee with Jeff's oldest sister Pat. Her husband, a minister, delivered the service during which the church choir performed "It Came upon a Midnight Clear." A couple of weeks later, Jeff asked Pat to look up the fourth verse of that song in her hymnal and to copy it for him in calligraphy. Not thinking too much of it, she did as he asked. After Jeff died, the family thought again of the words to that song and recited them at his funeral. It was these same lines that Jerry later transcribed onto the fabric panel in memory of his only brother.

46

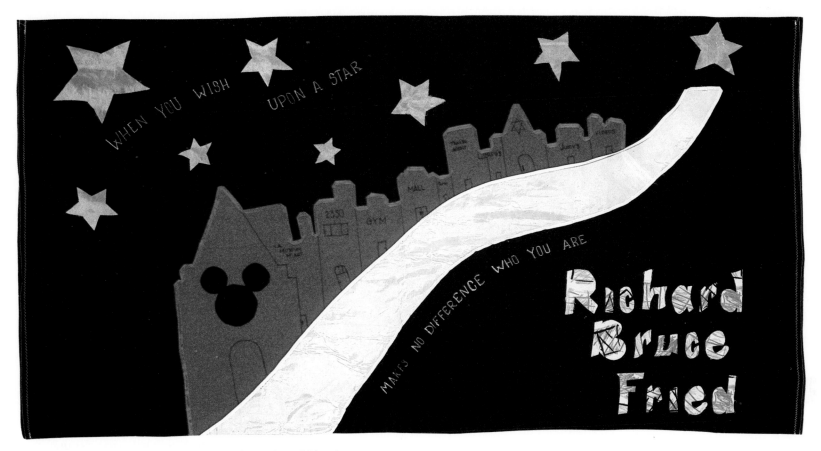

WHEN YOU WISH UPON A STAR

MAKES NO DIFFERENCE WHO YOU ARE

Richard Bruce Fried

Beca Kulinovich, a friend of Richard Fried and his sister Suzanne, created this panel. Suzanne shopped for the fabric, "but I couldn't handle making the quilt," she says.

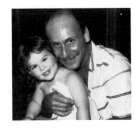

Richard with his niece Nicole on her first birthday.

My brother Richard had style. Richie always liked it when I showed up in "ELAY" dressed up and made up.

Richie owned more suits than anyone I ever knew, even our Dad. Richie was my birthday present when I was three years old; he was born on February 19, 1952, I was born on February 26, 1949. I loved to go dancing with Richie when the two of us lived in New York City and were enjoying our newfound freedom and pride as gay — we wondered for a long time if we were the only gay brother-sister act.

Richie loved life and life loved him back . . . he was creative in his field and working at Disney Studios seemed fitting. I still cannot walk into a video store without tears coming to my eyes, I never look in the direction of the cartoons and kid's movies, it is still too painful.

AIDS is the cruelest four-letter word I know. AIDS came into Richard's life and destroyed it.

AIDS is the cruelest four-letter word I know. AIDS stole my baby brother from me.

Suzanne R. Fried

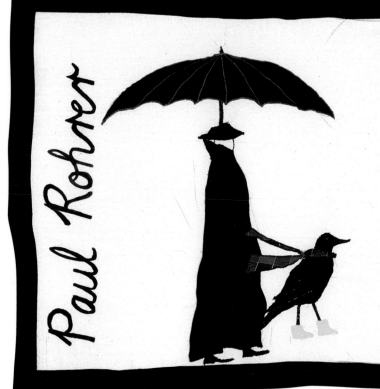

Last night it did not seem as if today it would be raining.

– Edward Gorey –

Paul Rohrer

Keith chose an Edward Gorey cartoon for Paul's panel because of its shock and surprise. "Just as things are going well, there is this," he says. "Who could have expected it?"

Paul Rohrer taught social studies at Edison Junior High School in Council Bluffs, Iowa, in 1969. He began teaching there the year after I had gone on to high school. However, he had my sister in his class and I frequently had afterschool conversations with him and my English teacher, Beth Reeves, when I visited there. This was during the Vietnam era and I was in a period of moral, ethical, political and personal searching. Though sexuality was not discussed, I was not surprised when I saw him at a gay bar in Omaha, Nebraska, during the summer I came out (1974). This was very important to me. I was not certain that I could be gay and still be everything else that I had come to know about myself. Paul was an example of a man with enormous personal integrity who was gay. My last conversation with him was when he visited St. Paul in 1984. We talked about the process that brought us from adult/child, teacher/student to being together as two equal adults. He died of AIDS in the winter of 1986.

Keith Gann

Keith Gann planned to make a difference in the world. He grew up in a working-class, fundamentalist Christian family of nine. Hunting and fishing were the things that boys did in his Iowa town. Keith, however, became an avid newspaper reader, a straight-A student, president of the student council and editor of the high school yearbook. He had his own ideas of what education should be. In high school, he formed an alternative study group in which members read Native American legends and explored gestalt therapy.

Keith owed much of his strong-minded, independent streak to the nurturing and encouragement provided by a few role models including Paul Rohrer. Paul's influence helped Keith, 33, decide to take on his life's work as a social worker, caring for mentally retarded adults and working for Child Protective Services in St. Paul, Minnesota.

Not long after hearing about Paul's death, Keith found that he, too, had AIDS. Keith entered the hospital with pneumocystis pneumonia in January 1987, having been diagnosed a year previously with ARC. He had lost a lot of weight and was scared. The same day he called home to tell his family that he had AIDS, his sister-in-law had a baby boy and they were celebrating the birth of this new child. His youngest brother was about to be married in February, so Keith's mother suggested that they put off telling the rest of the family about his diagnosis until after the wedding.

Keith discouraged his mother and sister from visiting him in the hospital because it has always been important to him that he look good in front of his family. Now it became urgent for him to speak with his family. "In the summer, I realized that I wanted to let them into my life more," he says. "I decided that I had to take the lead in order for them to get to know me again and to get to know what it's like for me living with this disease, and what it might be like for them."

In August, Keith went home to talk to his parents. He knew that they had not mentioned his AIDS diagnosis to anybody. He wanted to say to them, "Your secrecy makes me feel that you are ashamed of me. You are ashamed that I have AIDS and that I am gay. There is no time left for shame."

In trying to come up with a loving, creative way to broach the subject of his illness and his probable early death — something that they were not ready to deal with — Keith brought a project home. He had decided to make a quilt panel for his teacher, Paul Rohrer. "The idea was to make visiting my family a bit easier," Keith explains. "Sometimes they get bored, and this would give us something to do. It might open the door for us

to talk about my having AIDS. Because Paul was from Council Bluffs, I thought it would bring it closer to home."

As it turned out, the Ganns were fully engaged with canning and other harvest activities. "I really do understand that when the crops are in, you have to can, so I didn't take it personally," Keith says, laughing. "But I was disappointed. Bringing Paul's panel home didn't really accomplish what I had set out to do."

Nevertheless, Keith recruited other helpers. He asked his high school girlfriend, Cathy, and her mother to work on Paul's panel. Working in the basement at the home of Cathy's parents, they sewed into the night — four in the morning, to be exact, although Cathy's mom went to bed at about one. When Keith was first diagnosed, Cathy checked out a videotape about AIDS from the library for Keith's parents. She hoped it would help prepare them for what was ahead.

Keith wanted Paul's panel to salute the strength he had learned from the older man. "He had shown me some solid values, integrity, and concern about justice in the world," says Keith. "I had this fear that coming out as a gay man would just be glitter and glitz. Knowing Paul helped me realize that my sexuality would be one part of my life and would fit with everything else."

After a conversation with a reporter, Keith asked his mother if she would mind his story being included in an article about The Quilt.

"What if people turned against us?" she asked.

"Possibly one of your friends will see my name or face and associate me with AIDS or being gay," Keith told his mother. "If that happens, I'm really sorry if they treat you badly. But it's not your fault or my fault — it's their fault. I need to do this — speak out about AIDS — this is for us!"

"Go ahead. You'll do what you want to do anyway," she replied, reminding Keith of the way she used to respond when he nagged at her as a kid.

In fact, Keith decided to make a television commercial educating the public about safe sex, and he's editing a newsletter for people affected by AIDS called *PW Alive!*

Despite his scrupulous presentation as he laid out his need for total acceptance, his mother could not support him enthusiastically. Keith thought that she'd never understand until one day she explained a private anecdote from her own life. Ever since her children were little, she had sewn pillows, stuffed animals, quilts and clothes for them. She told him that she will always continue to make things despite her debilitating arthritis because she wants her children to have something to remember her by. "I suddenly felt kind of naked," says Keith. "It's one thing being able to look at the possibility of my own death, but to hear that expressed so openly by my mother caught me off guard. She did understand what I was talking about after all. The connection was so strong and so clear — how each of us are facing mortality — each other's and our own."

Although Keith's illness wasn't mentioned at his brother's wedding, everyone sensed that this could be their last time together. Relatives kept snapping photographs of Keith, and he knew exactly what was going on. This event had to be perfect. It was, after all, the first Gann wedding where there was no major family fight. When he was first diagnosed, Keith's greatest fear was that his brothers and sisters would not want him to be around their children. One of the joys of his trips home is the time he spends with his nieces and nephews.

"I'm letting my family know more than ever before who I am," says Keith. "The reality is that I do respect all of them, and myself, and have worked real hard to come to a place where I can be myself and maintain a relationship with them."

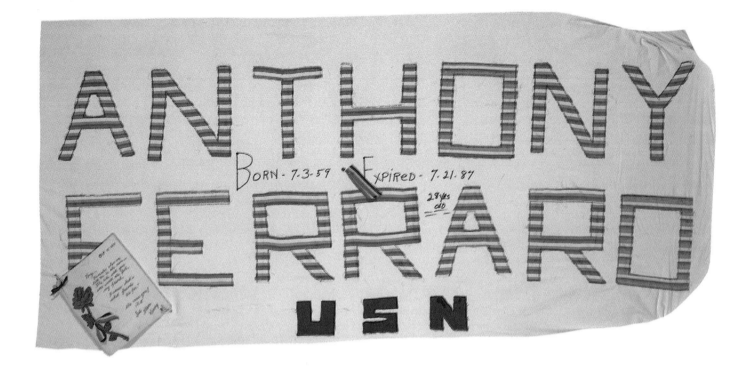

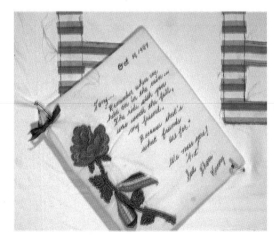

My son Anthony was discharged 18 months ago from the Navy — he loved the service and had a great love for his country. We stood by him to the end, a very courageous young man, we are very proud of him. So terrible a disease — so good a life is taken away. The cloth I made for my son is very meaningful as you can see — red, white and blue.

Ann Des Rosiers, 49, had never heard of AIDS until her son Anthony, then nine years into his navy career, called her from a Maryland hospital and asked, "Mom, could you take me home?" A few weeks later, Ann made the decision to leave her office job to look after Anthony full-time. In the two-family house she shares with her 25-year-old married daughter in Worcester, Massachusetts, Ann set up a room for her son, equipped with a hospital bed, a commode, a wheelchair, and an over-the-bed table.

Anthony's disease affected his brain and left him paralyzed and blind. With help from her mother, daughter and husband, Ann took care of Anthony for 18 months until he died in July 1987, shortly after his 28th birthday. As Anthony's illness progressed, home-care nurses helped Ann through the night. Now Ann has returned to school to study home care herself so that she can nurse other AIDS patients in their homes. She plans to work with the people who helped her look after her son.

"Worcester is a small city. Everything is hush-hush, and that's how we had to live it," Ann says. "People were very funny. We were isolated for 16 months. Even now I don't have people coming over. My mother and daughter were here every day, but I can count the friends I've seen on my fingers. I'm starting to spend time only with AIDS families now. I have nothing in common with anybody else."

All the materials Ann used for Anthony's quilt panel came from his bed. After a thorough washing of the linens, she stitched Anthony's name onto his red, white and blue pillow cases, along with the letters "U.S.N." Anthony's 52-year-old stepfather did all the cutting, and his 73-year-old grandmother took the fabric home for stitching because the Des Rosiers' sewing machine didn't work. Anthony's sister also joined in to help.

"He was my firstborn," Ann says. "He was my love."

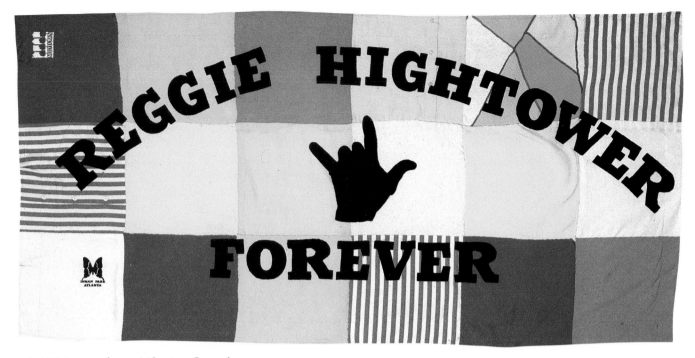

Art Peterson from Atlanta, Georgia, created this cloth memorial to honor his lover, 27-year-old Reggie Hightower.

Ours was a unique relationship. We had lots of obstacles which we overcame to make our relationship grow: He was deaf, I was hearing; He was black, I was white; We were both gay and proud. We agreed that these were the happiest times of our lives. We lived and shared a totally "married" life.

I don't have many ideas on how he should be memorialized—perhaps a carving on the side of Stone Mountain here in Georgia. I feel it's a shame that I can't convey to others how great a life he lived—for he left no mark to be forever immortalized except deep within those people he loved and those who loved him. How do I fully express his life to those who never met him? The memories are so wonderful and yet they cause so much pain.

His panel is composed of shirts that he wore—some his, some mine. They were hand-sewn (by me) with double thread and double sewn in places for strength and durability. Please display it prominently.

The handsign in the middle is sign language for "I Love You."

Sincerely, Art

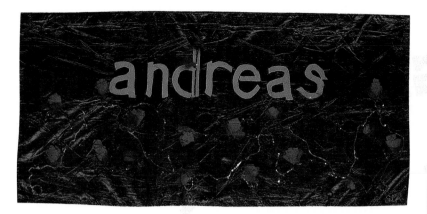

Scott Lago chose purple, the color of mourning, for the memorial he made to honor Andreas, a coworker at Neiman-Marcus. "He was a stately and proper man," says Scott. "He always held doors open for people."

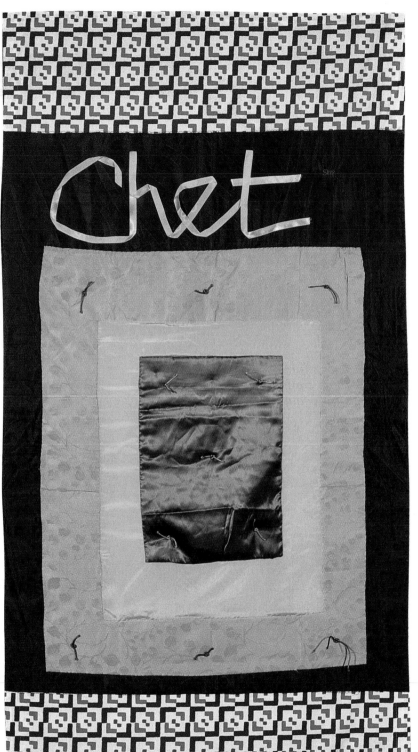

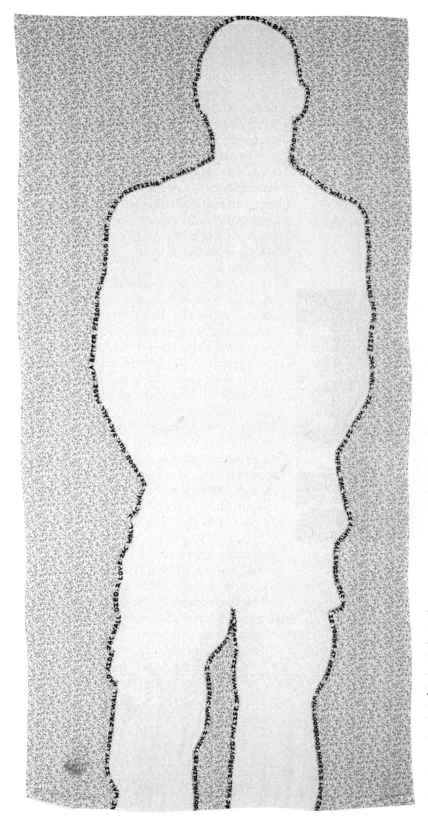

Every year, David Kemmeries gave his lover Jac Wall a portrait for Valentine's Day and his birthday. When Jac was very ill, he propped himself up against a wall so that David could trace his silhouette for one final portrait. "He had a hard time standing," remembers 27-year-old David, who has the same silhouette in red neon hanging on his living room wall. "From a distance you can see that it's a person," says David of The NAMES Project portrait, "but you have to get up close to read what he is really about."

There are 50,000 women who carry the AIDS virus. Not all of them are addicts; most of them are disadvantaged and all are capable of producing infants with AIDS.

Nancy was a friend, I loved her and her family. With all the pain we suffered in the year and a half I knew her, I still had fun. We ate together and laughed together and enjoyed being women and mothers together. We met wonderful people from the Task Force, caring physicians and nurses, self-sacrificing nuns and priests, sympathetic social workers. Nancy stands as a symbol of life for me, a defier of death, but she stands, too, for another, darker world. There are 50,000 potential Nancys and Boscos. Who will help them?

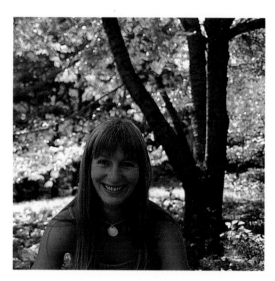

"Nancy carried on, sicker than I can imagine anyone being," says Hallie Wolfe (above), who entered Nancy's world of emergency rooms, evictions, soup kitchens and funeral plot arrangements, 18 months before Nancy died. "We will not stop AIDS," says Hallie, "until we deal with the poverty."

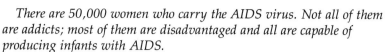

allie Wolfe was outraged when she first heard about physicians and nurses refusing to treat patients with AIDS. So during Christmas 1985, she decided to volunteer at the Mid-Hudson Valley AIDS Task Force in White Plains, New York. Hallie, a woodworker from Westchester County, says, "I thought I was going to be taking flowers and going to the theater with a gay man. To my horror, I was assigned to work with a woman who lives in the worst section of Yonkers. I had no idea what I was getting into."

Hallie spent 18 months as a "buddy" to Nancy, who was 26 and weighed 42 pounds when she died. Nancy's son, Bosco, died three months earlier. He was the second child she lost to AIDS-related complications. Nancy was not an intravenous drug user. The father of her first child was, and he probably infected Nancy with the AIDS virus. Bosco's father, a 19-year-old alcoholic, stayed with Nancy until the end. "We're not talking about AIDS alone," says Hallie. "We're talking about poverty. These people don't have enough to eat, a place to live or a job to support them. We will not stop AIDS until we deal with the other problems."

Although Hallie is taking a respite from the buddy program to be with her own family, she visits Nancy's 23-year-old sister and children often. Nancy's uncle has AIDS, her brother is a heroin addict, and her sister's baby has severe lymphadenopathy, a sign of immune abnormalities. "I feel like I am literally watching a family die," says Hallie.

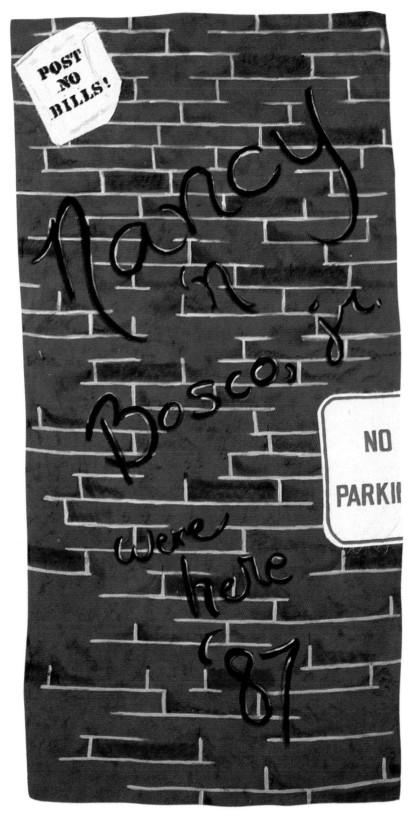

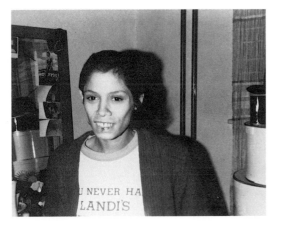

"She didn't want to die," says Hallie Wolfe of Nancy (above).

Nancy and her son Bosco, Jr., lived in a filthy, graffiti-covered neighborhood. While she was hospitalized, Nancy's landlord served her an eviction notice and spray-painted "Nancy, I always win!" on her apartment door. Hallie's 13-year-old daughter came up with the idea to write "Nancy and Bosco were here" across the wall they painted on this memorial panel.

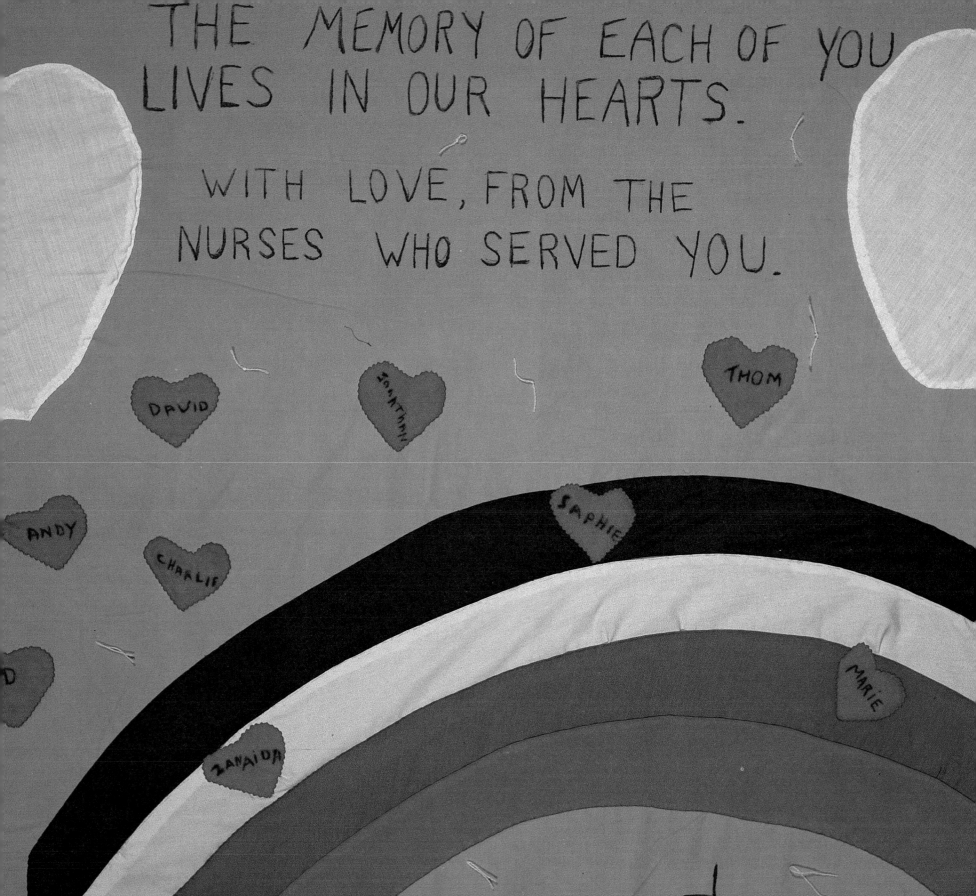

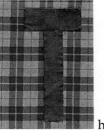he AIDS epidemic has brought out the best in many Americans. Thousands of "buddies" and home health-care attendants do grocery shopping, cooking and laundry, give massages, and care for the pets of people who do not have the strength to look after themselves. Children visit AIDS wards at Christmas, singing carols to cheer up the patients. Volunteers deliver free hot meals, and counselors provide people with AIDS, their families and lovers with emotional support. The gay community in particular has responded with tireless energy and compassion, but heroes have emerged from the straight community, too. People who have not had to cope with the reality of AIDS personally have come to the aid of strangers, helping them live through their last months with dignity.

The kindness of strangers has also shaped The Quilt: across the country, people have been moved to make panels in memory of people they never met. Nancy Kruh, a reporter with the *Dallas Morning News*, chose to make a panel for a man who died alone, and then wrote an article about what she was able to find out about the 25-year-old Texan. Richard Sumner from Chicago made a panel for Michael Murphy. Michael's mother is Richard's supervisor. "I didn't know Michael personally," says Richard. "I knew him through his mother's feelings of him. I decided to make Michael's panel not only in memory of him, but also as a tribute to his mother."

After *Newsweek* published a series of photographs profiling 302 people who had died of AIDS in one year, ending July 1987, panels arrived at The NAMES Project for many of the people that appeared in the piece. The article, titled "The Face of AIDS," prompted men, women and children across the country to make quilt panels for names and faces they had just learned of, including eight-year-old "Little Girl C" from Miami who, along with her two sisters, contracted AIDS through her mother; Amy Sloan, a 25-year-old mother from Indiana; six-year-old hemophiliac Layton Mullins from Marion, Ohio; Dominic Vasile, an intravenous drug user who lived on the streets in Boston; and two-year-old Jessica Hazard from Bloomington, Minnesota, who received a contaminated blood transfusion as an infant.

Some quilt panels reflect stories of extraordinary selflessness. Michael Lueders, a social worker who works with the elderly, made a quilt panel to honor 23-year-old Curt Norrup. Michael met Curt at the Los Angeles V.A. Hospital in March 1986, four months before Curt died. Curt had broken up with his lover and

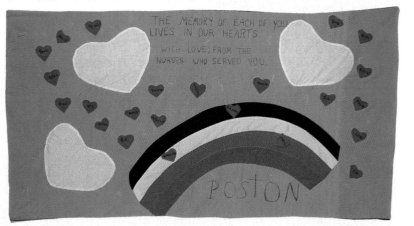

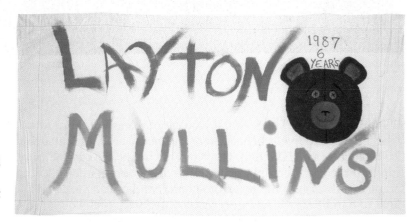

The photograph in Newsweek *of cherubic, smiling six-year-old Layton touched tenth-grader Rebecca Sweet who created this quilt panel in his memory.*

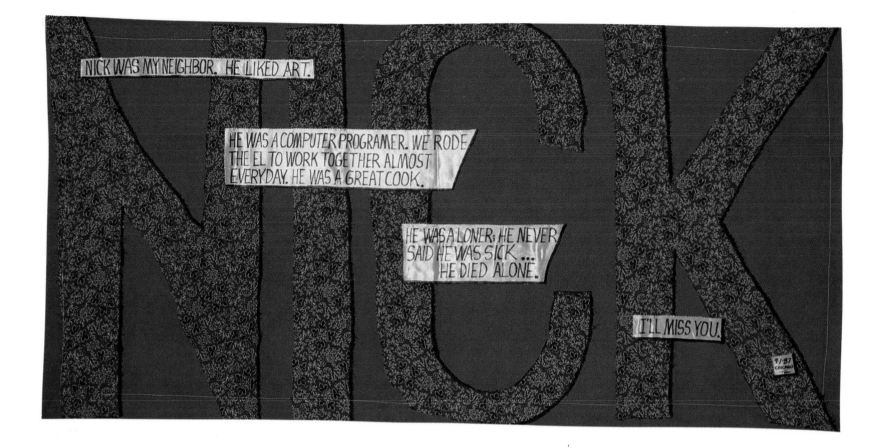

attempted suicide. The hospital would not release him until he found a place to live. Michael, who had never had any personal experience with AIDS, took Curt into his home and nursed him through the last months. Michael attended a seven-week class on home healthcare for the nonprofessional, and quickly learned how to handle Curt's seizures. "After Curt died, I felt so empty," says Michael. "I needed something to be completed so that his death was not in vain."

The quilt panel he made for Curt is simple — black cloth letters sewn onto gray fabric with pink elephants. "I spent 14 hours sewing with a lot of love and needle pricks," Michael writes, "but it was well worth it. I knew nothing of his life when I took him in, and because of that we became good friends. I pray that our short time together provided him some laughter and, hopefully, some joy."

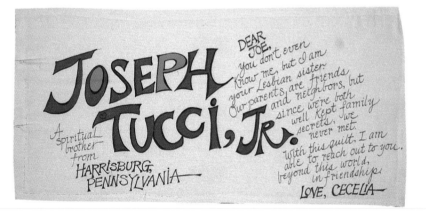

58

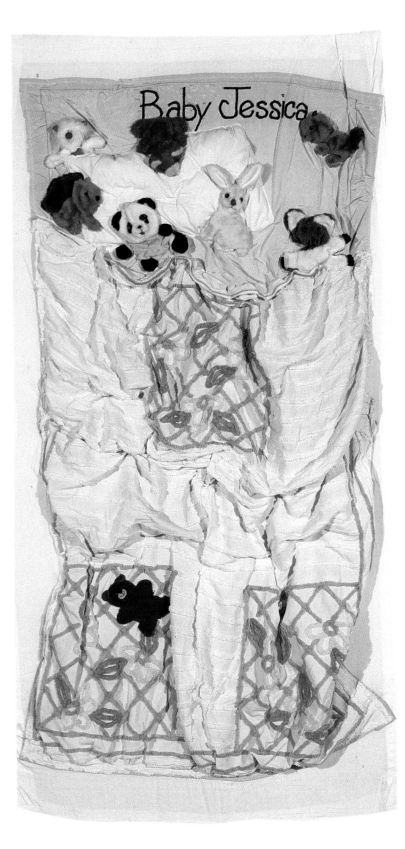

Kim Kubik and his girlfriend made this panel for Jessica Hazard, an infant who contracted AIDS from a contaminated blood transfusion. They were touched by her story, although they did not know the baby, and made this quilt in her memory.

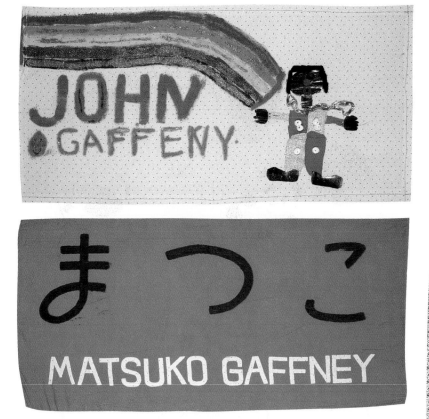

Barbara Cymrot and her lover Dafna Wu made this quilt to honor Matsuko Gaffney from Lowell, Massachusetts, who contracted AIDS from a tainted blood transfusion. She, in turn, infected her husband and her son.

Astar Lambert, a nine-year-old from San Francisco, created the panel for Matsuko's infant son, John, who was pictured in *Newsweek* because, she says, "I felt sorry for him."

Jean Hansen didn't know cellist Neal Lo Monaco personally, but she was moved by his music. "I wish I had told him of my appreciation of his artistic talent," she writes. "I miss him."

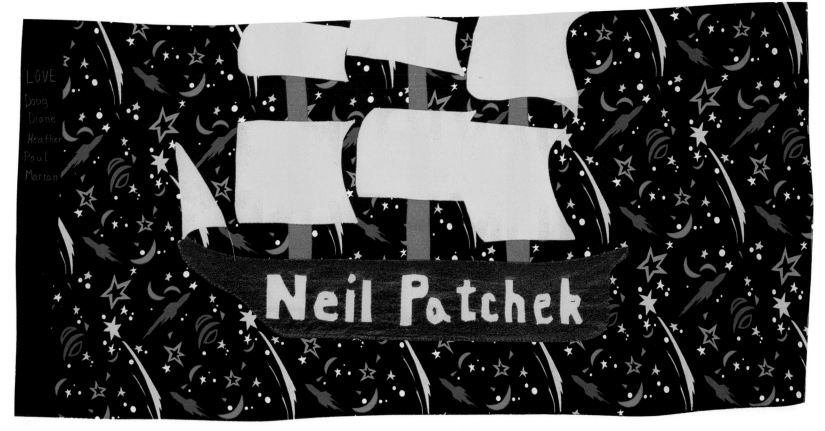

"I'm just a housewife," says 60-year-old Marian Mesner from Lincoln, Nebraska, who made this panel for a man who worked with her son in Denver. Although Marian did not know her son's friend very well, she felt compelled to make the panel. "I thought that there would be no recognition from his family," she says. "I felt bad about that. I feel bad about all the people who die of AIDS that nobody knows."

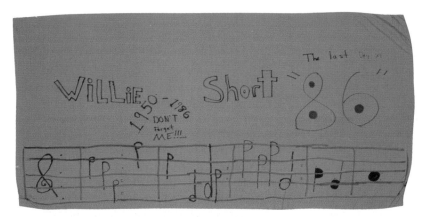

NAMES Project volunteer, 12-year-old Willi "Jack" Heard created this quilt panel in memory of Willie Short, a dishwasher from Houston. Willie's photograph was included in Newsweek's "The Face of AIDS" article along with his words, "Don't forget me. Mention my name now and again."

DAVID R. THOMPSON

1949-1986

avid Thompson worked as a librarian at Stanford University. A week after he died, each of his coworkers at Stanford's Green Library — about 300 people — received his prearranged gift: a single, long-stemmed yellow rose accompanied by a personal note.

It was this gentle farewell that prompted one colleague's remembrance to David. "This gesture made my day," says R. T. Carr, who never knew David but wrote a poem in his memory after receiving a rose. As a library portal monitor, R. T. checks the identification of everyone who enters the library, and probably saw David Thompson many times.

Someone sent me a flower!
This solitary yellow rose, done up
so meticulously, with obvious care.
I put 2 + 2 together and suddenly it
*   equaled 4.*
I remembered, a quiet note in the Library
*   Bulletin.*
A memorial service.
A man, one year younger than my age,
struck down by a terrible disease,
a leaf pulled down way too early,
brought even closer to us because he was one of
*   our own.*
Yet, sadly now because he touched me with his
*   rose,*
I don't believe I ever met him. If I did,
I hope I smiled at him.
*   R. T. Carr*

David's parting gift also found its way onto a quilt panel created for David by the Green Library staff, who held a lunchtime sewing circle in the library conference room. A bright yellow felt rose appears prominently alongside University pennants. "Through our common concern for David, the Stanford libraries became a very much more human place," says music cataloger Beth Rebman. "In facing the terrible tragedy of his illness and in discussing what it meant to us, we all began to talk to each other, and learned to know each other in a new and more complete way than we did before."

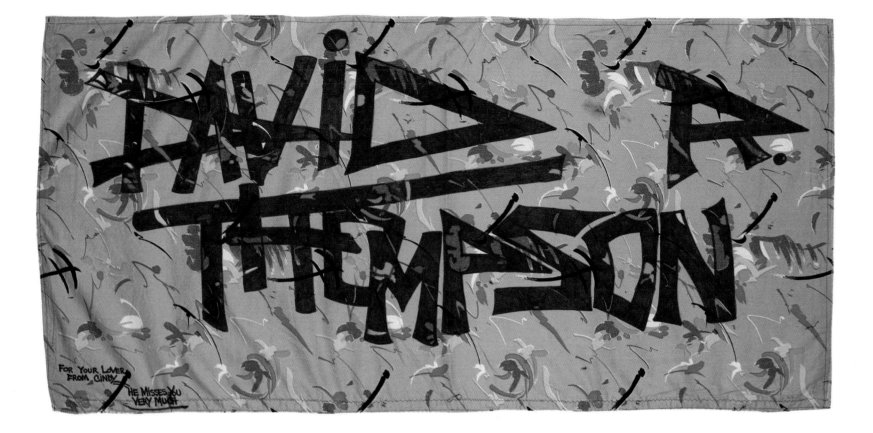

Another panel for David Thompson came from a more distant source.

I did not know David Thompson or his lover. I had no photograph to part with or any fond memories of his experiences. We were strangers. But when he died I felt a loneliness that scared me beyond belief. On October 23, 1986, I came upon his death notice in the paper. It read:

"On Sunday evening, October 12, my lover and best friend David R. Thompson, died of AIDS. It was a wonderful ten years. I will miss him very much."

This letter is to David's lover in the hopes that he will realize that his love for David reached out and touched my heart so tenderly . . . so tenderly.

Dear David's Lover,

Please know my intent, when making this panel, was not to invade your memories or life with David. I have no memories to share of him but I do share one thing with you. On October 23, 1986, a pain went through my heart that was unbearable. A loneliness for the loss of a complete stranger — a potential friend. To this day I cry when I think of how you must miss each other.

You see, I had to know his name would be among the others. To be seen by his friends and the friends he would have had. Also this panel has released some of my pain for David. A very confusing pain for me because I have never loved a complete stranger.

Love, Cindy

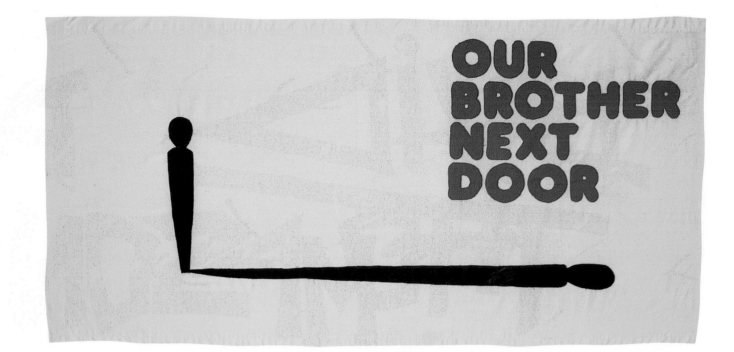

ayne Hadley's landlord told him that a man dying of AIDS was moving in next door with his mother. Wayne doesn't remember if he ever saw this neighbor, but does know that he felt a deep need to memorialize him.

Wayne designed a yellow horizontal banner with a single figure in silhouette on one side, and a shadow running along the bottom. In purple lettering, he wrote "Our Brother Next Door." "Once I decided to do it, the banner just kind of made itself," says Wayne, a Cincinnati schoolteacher. "While I was making it, I felt very private — it was a real personal thing."

I'd sit on the couch and gaze out my bay window at his window and wonder what he was doing. I'd wonder if maybe he was sitting at his bay window thinking about his life and dying, and wonder if he was frightened. And then I'd get frightened and angry and then just wait — and I knew he was doing the same. So in this memorializing banner I needed to say something for him and for all of us that know the fear of uncertainty.

With love and fear, Wayne M. Hadley

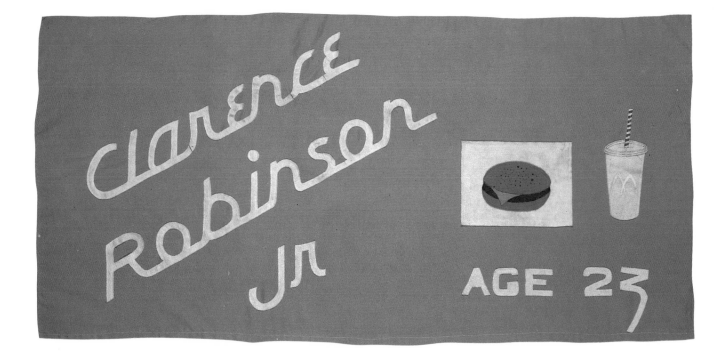

"My friends told me about a 23-year-old who was quite seriously ill with AIDS," writes 54-year-old Sonny, a retired businessman from Lakeland, Florida. *"He was in the county hospital and was not being given any treatment. He was placed in an open hallway, and everyone avoided him, except one gay nurse. The only family member who came to see him was his divorced father. It was truly a shock to see this burly, rough-cut, unskilled phosphate-mine worker as he talked (and cried) about the mistreatment of his son. This man had tried every possible way to get medical help for his son."*

Sonny found it impossible to forget the cruel treatment of AIDS patient Clarence Robinson, Jr. So in 1986, he and his wife Mary decided to take action. They joined the Polk AIDS Support Services (PASS) in Polk County, Florida, a volunteer group that runs a hot line and works with people with AIDS. Sonny started attending PASS meetings strictly out of compassion, having no idea that in April 1987 he, too, because of a tainted blood transfusion six years earlier, would be diagnosed with AIDS. "I didn't fit the AIDS profile," Sonny says. "My doctors did not test me for AIDS at first because I am an older, married man. People need to know how widespread the disease has become." Joined by their son and daughter-in-law, Sonny and Mary responded by increasing their volunteer work and becoming active AIDS treatment lobbyists, writing letters to Congress and to Nancy Reagan.

Now Sonny and Mary spend most of the year at a country home in rural North Carolina. "Our neighbors are so backward and uneducated about AIDS," says Sonny. "They're still living in the eighteenth or nineteenth century."

While teaching their community about AIDS, Sonny and Mary have made four quilt panels, including one for Clarence Robinson, Jr. They never met Clarence, but they heard how he fought his loneliness by devising ways to prolong the visits of the support service volunteers. He would ask visitors to bring him a Coke and a hamburger from the local MacDonald's, and then beg them to stay until he finished eating. In Clarence's honor, Sonny and Mary stitched a felt hamburger next to his name on his fabric memorial.

Sonny and Mary are at work on their fifth quilt panel. "We sew and then we cry and then we hold each other," says Sonny. "But it is important to have some type of commemoration."

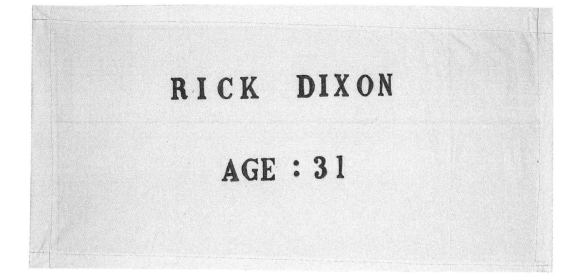

RICK DIXON

AGE : 31

My son's battle with AIDS began in January 1984. A small lesion on his nose proved to be the dreaded KS.

We went through many changes over the course of the disease. In the beginning, when he was part of a study down at the N.I.H. in Bethesda, we were so hopeful! The first two years of his illness were "good" years. Rick was concentrating on living with AIDS.

Then came a period of overwhelming depression. That was such a sad time for us all. There were brief periods when the disease affected his mental status. This, to him, was the scariest of all.

By May of 1986, my son asked to come live with me. He no longer had the energy to even prepare his own food. I was glad to be able to be there for him. By October 1986, I found it necessary to resign from my position as a kindergarten teacher to be available on a full-time basis for my son. I found strength I didn't know I had as we progressed toward the more debilitating stage of his illness. I have the comfort of knowing that my special care kept him alive as long as possible, with the hope that something would surface that could make a difference. We lost that chance, but we're determined to continue to do what we can to see that those now struggling fare better.

The last five or six weeks of his life had an abundance of beauty in it: he allowed many of his old friends and new ones in. We all shared our mutual love — and grief with him. . . .He became more venturesome.

One of the things that happened was he rediscovered an old restaurant he'd once enjoyed with a special friend. We became befriended by Martha Mosler, a waitress who made him feel like a king. She ignored his wasted body and facial lesions and gave him star treatment every time we appeared. He always consumed a full-course meal there — at a time when eating was routinely difficult for him. His doctor confirmed that this waitress really made a difference!

I'm so grateful for those beautiful last days! My son had not been an easy patient for a long time. He was so helpless, so he exerted power by complaining. I knew what was going on intellectually, but that didn't keep the treatment he was venting from hurting. (I was glad, though, that he felt free enough to attack me and that he wasn't turning it inward.)

As I said, the final memories, when he was at peace for the most part, I wouldn't trade for anything. He returned to his loving, appreciative former self.

It's been five weeks now. Much of the time I'm still numb with grief. I know the hard part is to come. I haven't truly accepted the finality of his death.

This quilt means so much to me and to those whose lives my son's touched. When I saw all the panels, I was tempted to take mine back and add more to it. Then I said, "No, Deane. You and your 82-year-old friend, Hilda, spent a wonderful afternoon and evening together creating a very simple panel that was carefully printed with your son's name and the message: "age: 31." Rick was a very private person. This is perhaps enough to say in public — cut down before he had a chance to find out what his potentials really were. A lot of time and love went into that simple panel. Better, now, that you go on with things that need your attention." And so I submitted it as is.

Lovingly yours,
Deane Dixon (Rick Dixon's Mom)

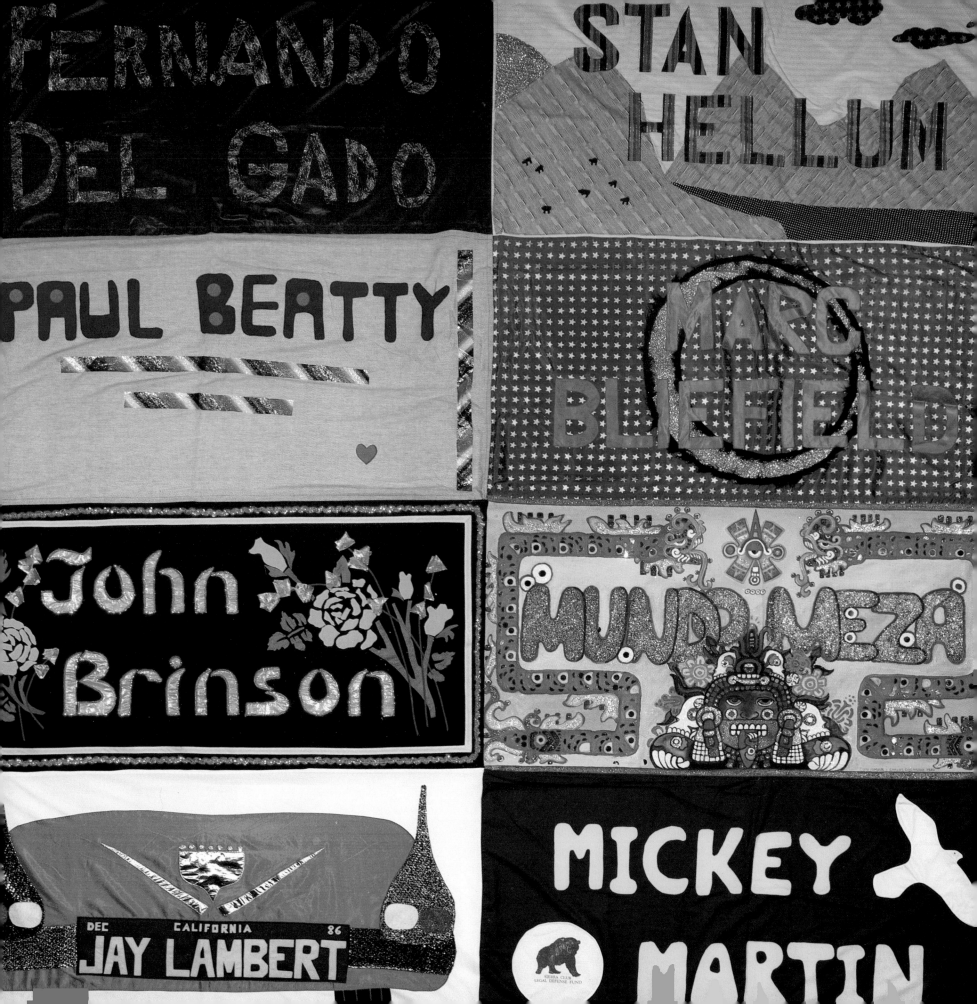

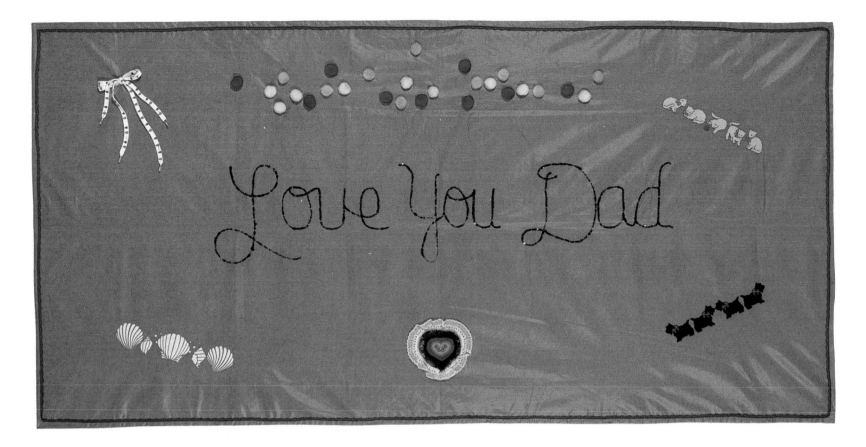

rla Ellsworth thought she had a typical suburban marriage. John, her husband of 22 years, was a lawyer and vice-president of a church-oriented insurance group in Washington, D.C. He traveled frequently, but that, too, was typical. Sometimes she wished that there was more "togetherness" in their marriage, but then, so did all her friends.

Arla's perception of her world turned upside down on June 10, 1986, when the family doctor called to inform her that her husband was dying of AIDS. They had just spent ten days vacationing together in Hawaii. John hadn't told her that he was sick. Five days after their return he was hospitalized, and Arla learned for the first time that he had AIDS meningitis. Six months later he was dead.

Arla wanted to believe that John contracted AIDS from a blood transfusion, but she knew very well that he had never had one. "First there was this numbness," she says. "I didn't want it to penetrate. I didn't want to know that John was gay. I couldn't deal with the stigma and the betrayal. But I knew that I was going to have to face it. I tried, I didn't know too much then, to talk to John about the fact that I realized that he was bisexual." John responded with denials that he had AIDS. He also denied that he had sex with men.

John was in the hospital for six weeks, and Arla visited him every day. Their children visited, too. Arla told the children, a son in college and a daughter in high school, that their father had AIDS. Nevertheless, John's denials persisted. "John didn't want to talk," Arla remembers. "The kids didn't want to talk. I didn't know what to do. Nobody wanted to talk. It was like a nightmare."

Arla didn't know how to care for John when he came home from the hospital. "Do you need to wear gloves and gown up like the nurses do?" she wondered. She didn't know if she could sit on the bed. "I needed to know more than how much Clorox and water you mixed to clean things," she says. "I needed to know how to relate day to day."

While John was still in the hospital, Arla attended her first AIDS Support Group meeting where she met Randy Reichart, a 24-year-old art student with pneumocystis. "Randy was blond and fair and hardly had to shave," Arla remembers. She was the only woman in the room, as well as the only straight person. "I went to strangers — people I thought that I'd never rub shoulders with — for support," she says.

Arla invited Randy, his brother Allen and Allen's lover Didier for dinner soon after John got out of the hospital. "John and Randy were the only people we — the kids and me — knew who had AIDS," says Arla. "To all be sitting at the table in our backyard, breaking bread together, was the closest we, as a family of four, got to acknowledging that John had AIDS. This would be the most open we could be about it. Randy asked John how he got AIDS, and once again John replied that he wasn't sure that he actually had AIDS."

After John died in November 1986, Arla still felt hurt and betrayed. Sometimes she questioned how much he really loved her. Because John refused to deal with his prognosis, Arla had to attend to all the papers in his estate after he died. She found letters confirming his gay life. "I was always pushing for more intimacy," she says. "He had led me to believe that I was enough," she recalls. "Now I know for a fact that I could never be enough." What kept going through her mind over and over again was, "If he cared about me at

all, how could he have put me at risk? He never did anything to protect me. Of all the people in my life, how could this person, my husband, be dangerous to me?" Arla has since tested negative for HIV antibodies.

In her mind, Arla knew that she wanted to forgive John, but she couldn't bring herself to think about their good times together. "Will my heart always be a rock?" she wondered. "When will I be able to feel again?"

Allen Reichart encouraged her to make a commemorative panel for John to be included in The NAMES Project quilt. Arla's 17-year-old daughter didn't want her father's name on the quilt. "It would make me uncomfortable," she admits. "I don't want people to be nasty to me and my friends." So in black glitter, in the space where the name should be, she simply wrote "Love you Dad."

Making the quilt helped Arla remember some of the happy times with John again. The shoelaces she sewed into it are for hiking and the green around the heart is for Christmas, two of John's great loves. She also attached a bit of the purple fabric from Randy Reichart's memorial panel around the heart. Their 21-year-old son, a business major, ironed on the decals, and Arla's mother helped put the panel together.

A full year after John's death, Arla went to the cemetery. She lay on his grave, wanting to be close to him, and cried. "I'm no longer crying because I'm mad at what you have done to me," she said. "I'm crying out of love and forgiveness. What a lonely life you must have had, John, not really knowing who you were.

"It's almost Christmas. I can't believe that you are not here to cut down our tree and stop for coffee, just as we always do. Christmas together, making love in front of the fireplace. I want to be near you. I want to be with you. I want you back.

"Now I feel like other people, mourning someone I loved so much," says Arla. "Now I can say, 'I love you for you, who-

ever you were. I love you for all you gave to my life.' There was pain for me that John was dishonest, but then I think of the joy that John had from having children. I wouldn't want to deprive him of that. I was married to him and I've got these two beautiful kids.

"I had a driving need to stay with people with AIDS and people who are gay. The men in my support group helped me get acquainted with a side of John I didn't know — the giving, caring side of the gay personality. I'm lucky that there are men who have been willing to open themselves to me.

"I never thought that I'd be in the minority with a bunch of gay people," Arla says. "I wanted to find out about AIDS, but I have learned so much more. Some nights I can't sleep. Thoughts about the inhumanity of our society are racing through my mind. I've been a guest in the homes of gay people. I've gone to their parties. I'd grown to love them. It's ridiculous that I'm O.K. in this society and they are not."

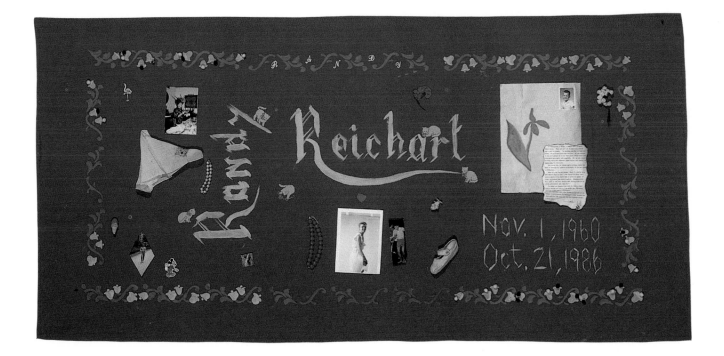

llen Reichart glued so many decals and trinkets to his brother's panel that it seems as if the contents of the bottom drawer of a bureau have spilled out onto the fabric. Amidst the mementos is a Mickey Mouse for the years that Randy worked as a teacher's aide at a preschool, a page of doodles from Randy's sketch pad, a clown from Randy's clown collection, a crystal for his interest in the supernatural, and costume jewelry for the great fun Randy always took in dressing up. The cloth cats attached with Velcro to the panel represent Randy's three pets — Miss Ruby, Zsa Zsa and Jake. They live with Allen now.

In his early 20's, Randy was a jet-setting student at the Corcoran School of Art in Washington, D.C. He loved to dance and party with the fast ultra-cool crowd. But when Randy became increasingly ill, his life-style slowed and his friends stopped coming by.

Allen, a 32-year-old nurse in a bone-marrow transplant ward, worried about his brother's persistent cough and high fevers. Allen took Randy to the hospital and was with him when Randy found out that he had AIDS. After the diagnosis, Randy then moved in with Allen and Allen's male lover, Didier. Soon Didier, a trade representative, opened up their two-bedroom town house for weekly support group meetings for people affected by AIDS.

Taking care of Randy was an emotional strain on Allen. "He was my brother — someone I grew up with — and I saw him deteriorating day by day," Allen says. "It was in some ways the same as taking on a child."

Allen asked his father and his four brothers and sisters to help him care for Randy, but family members made only occasional visits and then only after much pleading. Randy wrote each of them a personal letter asking, "Why are you deserting me while I am dying?" It was Allen who called the rest of the family at

3:30 A.M. the morning when Randy died.

The only acknowledgment Allen received was a thank-you note in the mail. "It was like a slap in the face," he says. "I'd gone through the most emotional experience in my life. Not only did they not inquire about Randy, but they never asked me how I was holding up either."

Allen suspects that his family blames him for Randy's wild, gay life-style, and think that ultimately he is responsible for Randy's AIDS and death. Nonetheless, Allen wrote to them and asked if they'd like to help make Randy's memorial quilt. There was no response.

"Making his panel made me feel that I was doing something for his honor," Allen says. "I'm not ashamed of him the way my family was." In the center of the panel, Allen glued a copy of the dedication he delivered at Randy's memorial service, and singed the edges of the paper "for the many friends and family that seemed to forget about him."

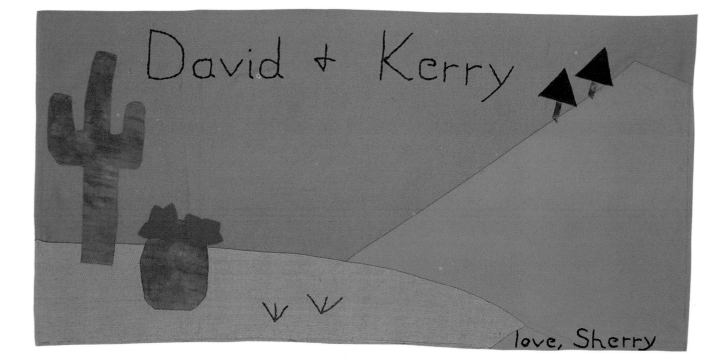

herry painted this panel for her brother, David, and his lover. Kerry died on January 21, 1987. David, his life partner and best friend, died three weeks later.

This quilt represents David and Kerry's love for the desert and mountains of Arizona. David loved cactus in bloom. Kerry owned a little land at the top of a mountain. I thought about putting in something very funny because of David and Kerry's sense of humor, but this is what I finally decided on.

In this quilt everything is paired in twos because they were together, and are together in all.

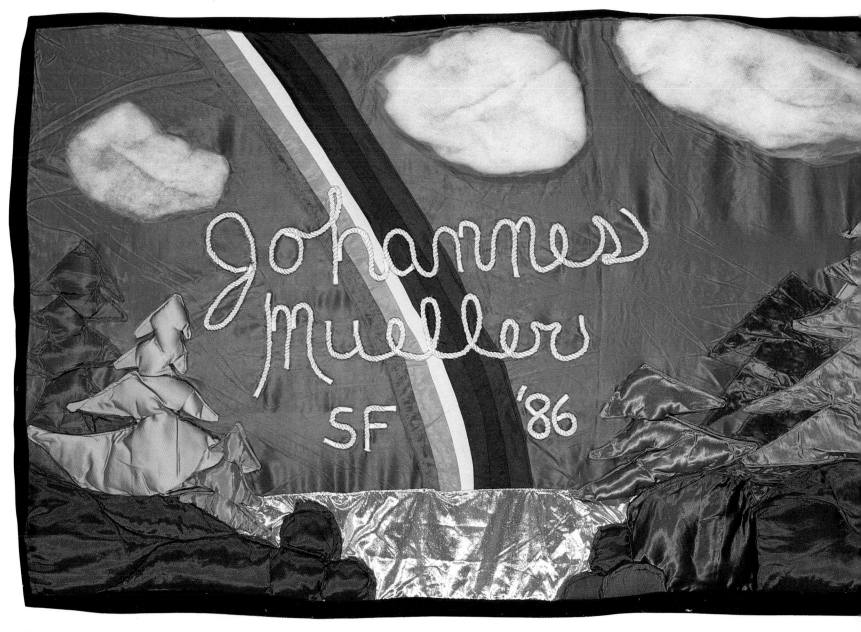

"Oh Joh, I love you so!" writes Robert Bowling, Johannes's lover of 14 years. In 1967, Johannes moved from Munich, Germany, to San Francisco, where he started his own electric company.

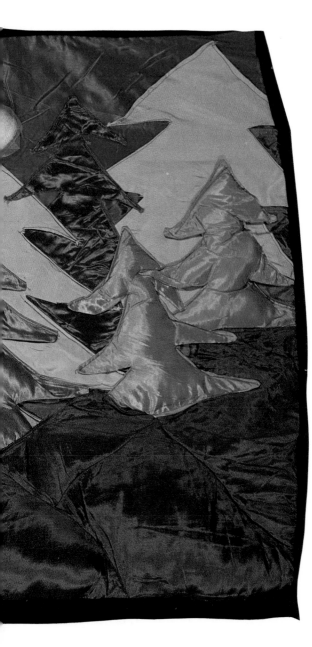

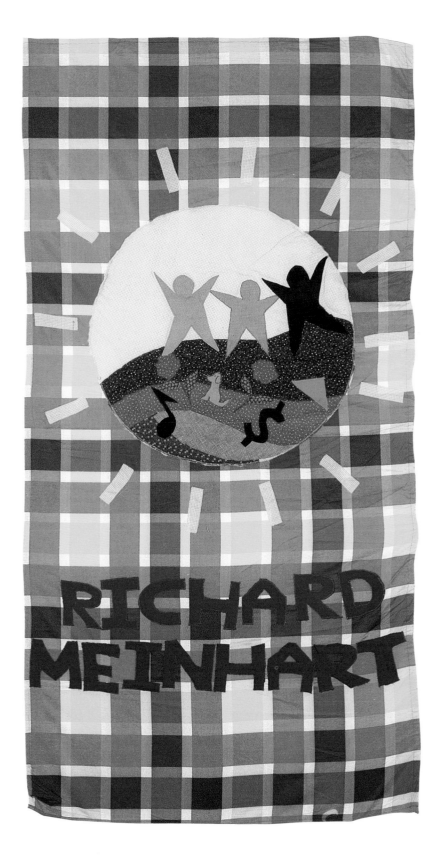

RICHARD MEINHART

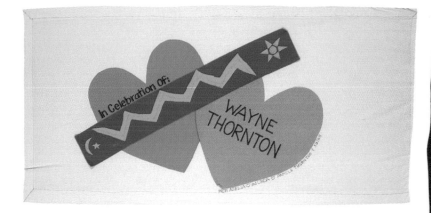

"Wayne was the father I never seemed to have," writes Pamela Thornton of San Anselmo, California, of her oldest brother, an FAA radar controller. "Our family was very poor and our father was rarely around. Wayne died in my arms and I will never feel the same again."

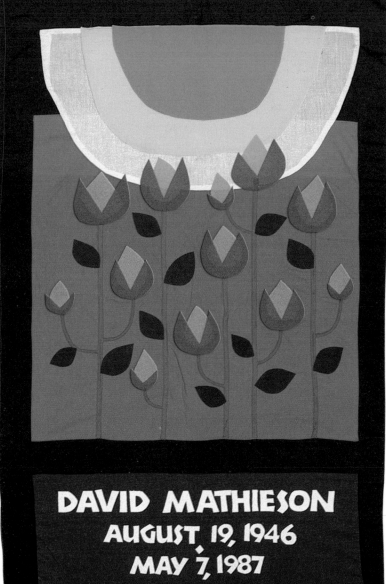

David Rile commissioned his ex-lover, graphic artist Karl Reque from Denver, to create this memorial for travel agent David Germann and ordained minister David Mathieson. "I lost my two best friends," says David Rile, "and I miss them so very much."

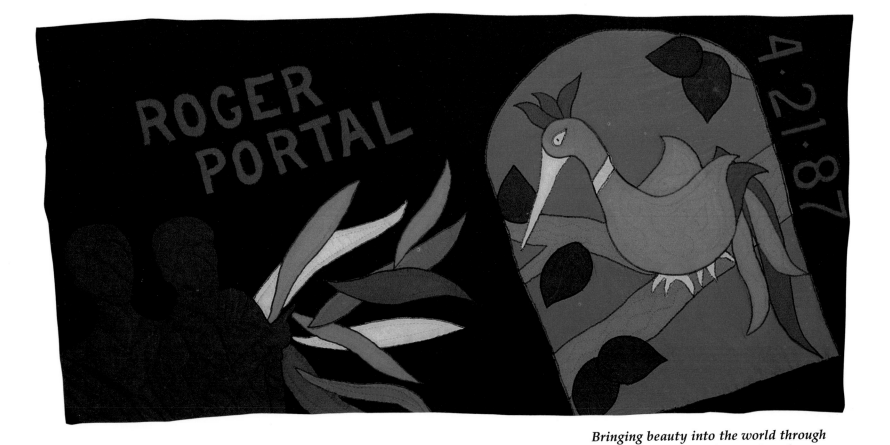

Bringing beauty into the world through his poetry, stained glass and garden were very important to 33-year-old Roger Portal from Boston. But it was his 14-year relationship with Steven Shuman, which ended with Roger's death from AIDS-related complications, that was his greatest source of pride.

Gary's mother made this panel for her 34-year-old son, a bird-watching enthusiast with red hair. She included names of his closest friends in the panel.

75

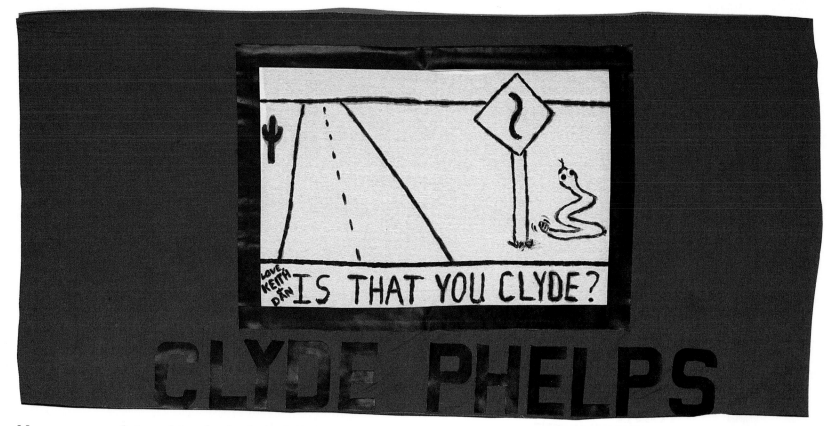

IS THAT YOU CLYDE?

Many young people turned to school principal Clyde Phelps for direction. "He was, and is, such a guiding force in our lives," says law student Dan Kane who created this panel with Keith MacPherson in Clyde's honor. "We still ask ourselves," says Dan, "Clyde, is that you?"

The heaviest panel in The Quilt, a three-by-six-foot slab of leather, was made for Mark Metcalf who arrived at U.C. Berkeley on a football scholarship and graduated with a Ph.D. in soil microbiology. "He showed his friends that you can explore all sides of yourself," says Environmental Protection Agency colleague Sue Schectman. "In the day he could be seen in a powder-blue seersucker suit meeting with farmers in the Central Valley discussing the Kesterson Reservoir pollution problem. At night he'd look like the Road Warrior, ready for anything." Once the all-American boy — captain of the football team, and date of the homecoming queen — Mark took his own life on July 4, 1986.

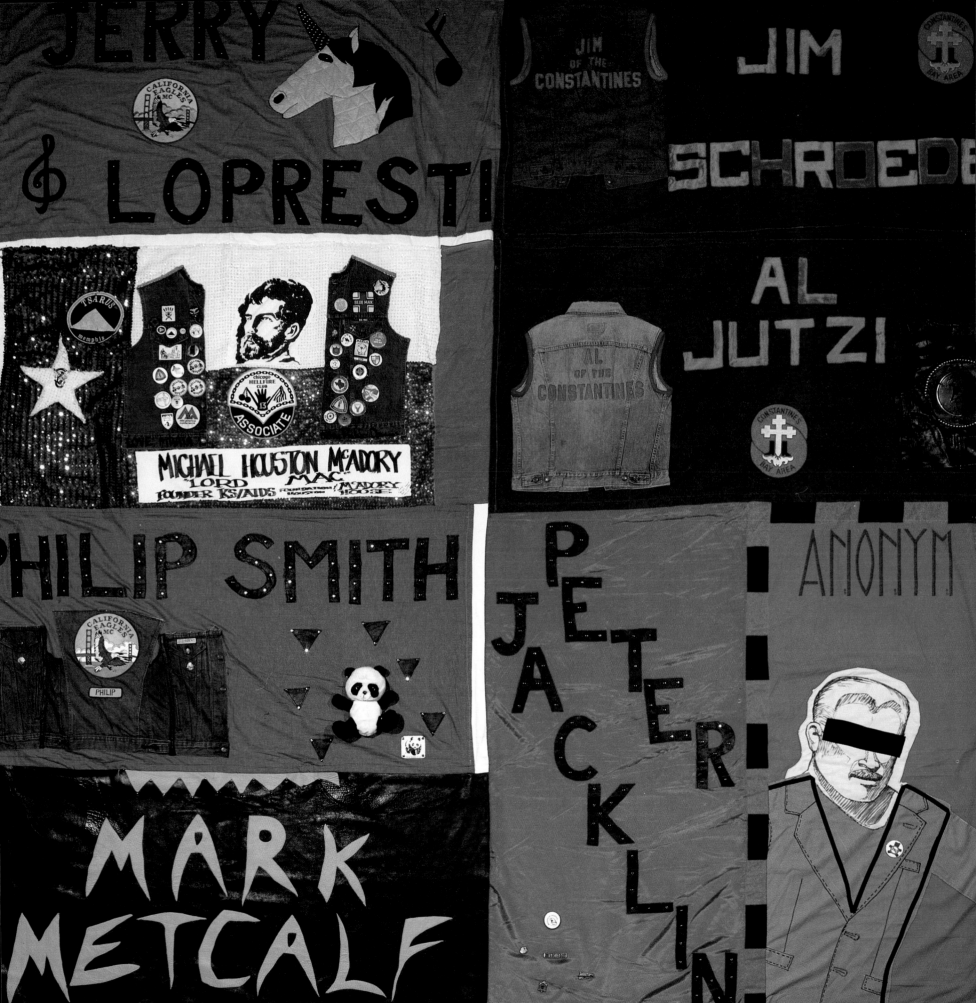

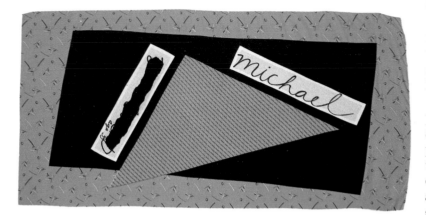

A man delivers a sky-blue panel with a pink triangle emblazoned on a swatch of black fabric for his lover. The name "Michael" is written on one side, but on the other side where his last name should appear, there is a gaping hole. His surname was cut out, literally, by his parents, when Michael's lover showed them the memorial he had made for their son.

AIDS has brought out the best in some Americans — an outpouring of compassion in response to a tragic reality. But society also makes outcasts of people suffering with AIDS. All too often, people with AIDS are shunned by their friends, alienated from their families and abandoned by the world. Families like the Rays of Arcadia, Florida, have been hounded out of their hometown after the neighbors discovered that the Rays' three hemophiliac sons were carrying the AIDS virus.

"I realize that this is The NAMES Project, but I must ask you one favor — please keep my friend anonymous," a woman writes. "I want to respect the privacy of the living. His parents and brother would be completely undone if they knew about this memorial. They maintain that he died of meningitis, not AIDS."

Meningitis, cancer, pneumonia, a rare blood disease — so many continue to maintain that their loved ones did not die of AIDS. The disease is still an embarrassment to some, who attempt to conceal the truth through the falsification of death certificates. Press spokesmen for Liberace, conservative fundraiser Terry Dolan, and clothing designer Perry Ellis tried to cover up their AIDS diagnoses. Lawyer Roy Cohn claimed he had a liver disease, the director-choreographer Michael Bennett had heart problems. Meanwhile, the families of people who have died of AIDS continue to live with their secret. A sister writes: "Jimmy was very handsome, but I haven't sent you his picture because my mom still has so much to deal with on this. She can't tell all her friends the truth."

Letters like this one arrive regularly at The NAMES Project, not for shame but for fear. "Three children were burnt out of their home," says one fearful mother. "I live in a small town," says another. "The neighbors are already suspicious." One mother nursed her son at home for two years, yet she had the local newspaper list cancer as the cause of his death in his obituary. Another mother, who writes, "My darling son was special! His specialness might be the very reason he was with us for such a short time — 27 years. God needed him more than we did. I am so very proud that he was my son," didn't put her son's full

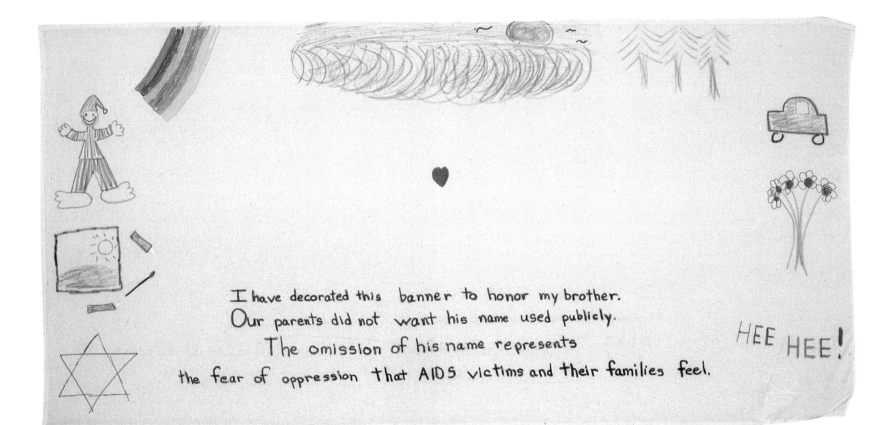

I have decorated this banner to honor my brother.
Our parents did not want his name used publicly.
The omission of his name represents
the fear of oppression that AIDS victims and their families feel.

HEE HEE!

name on the panel, respecting his wishes to keep his diagnosis a secret. As each panel-maker writes the name on a quilt, they are fighting that secrecy — a battle some gay people know well, having lived portions of their lives closeted. Many lovers grieve alone, worried that they may lose their jobs or their insurance if it becomes public knowledge that their partner died of AIDS. One man has been challenged with a lawsuit and a threat to run him out of town by his lover's family after they saw his panel in a newspaper article.

"Out of all those people who loved Ric and attended his funeral, only a handful knew that he died of AIDS," writes his lover, Paul Hill, from Dallas, Texas. "Being gay and having lived a lie, it was no problem lying about death as well. My lover who died of pneumocystis quickly became a roommate who died of viral pneumonia. This sham angers me now, but during that period of vulnerability which occurs immediately after a great loss, one can be talked into just about anything. This scenario repeats itself many times a day all over the United States. There are just too many people who don't realize that this awful disease already has touched their lives."

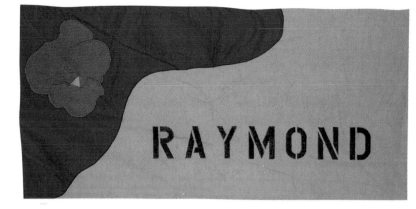

RAYMOND

"We omitted Raymond's surname," write Mark Shoofs and Sam Meaker, Raymond's practical and emotional support counselors, *"not only because his family would have been deeply disturbed to have Ray identified publicly in a gay context, but also because Ray himself never fully came out of the closet. Through his 66 years of life, this penumbra never quite lifted. Ray was alone in this world. We, his Shanti volunteers, listened to Ray and acknowledged his dignity. And when we listen to him now, in the silence of memory, we acknowledge it again."*

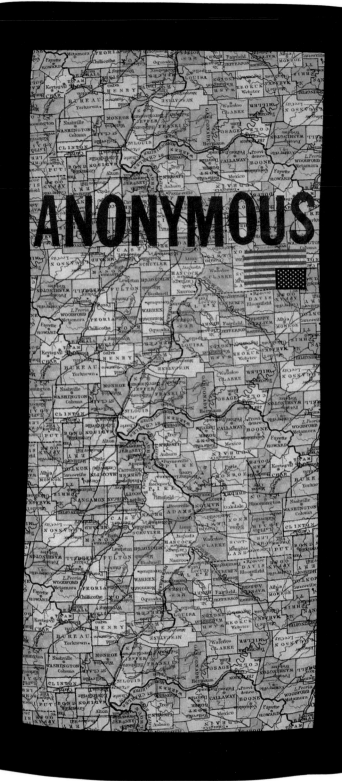

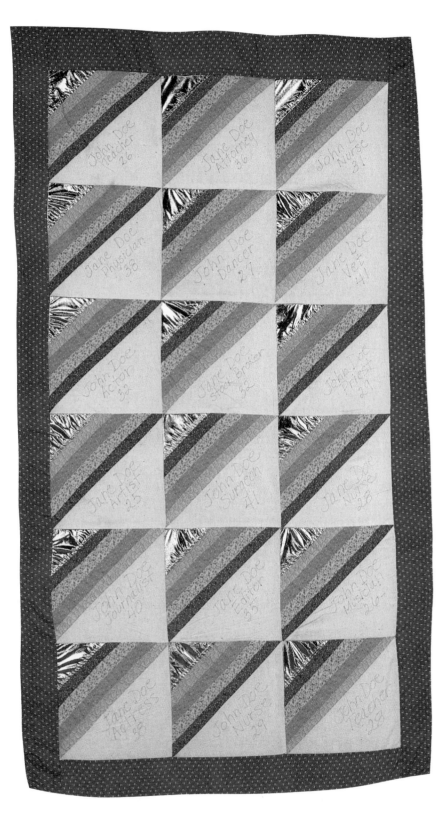

"So much of the straight community has looked away from this devastating disease," says JoAnne Melody, a 50-year-old medical transcriber from San Mateo, California. "This can't be done anymore. We need to become involved." JoAnne, a longtime quilter, designed her John and Jane Doe panels in a classic American quilt pattern to honor those who have died of AIDS but whose death certificates have been falsified.

Patty, whose family requested that her last name be withheld, contracted AIDS from a transfusion while having her wisdom teeth removed when she was 16 years old. She died six years later.

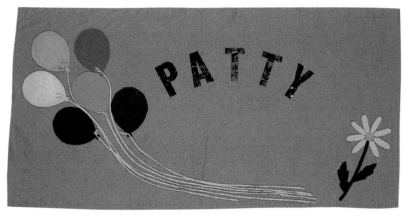

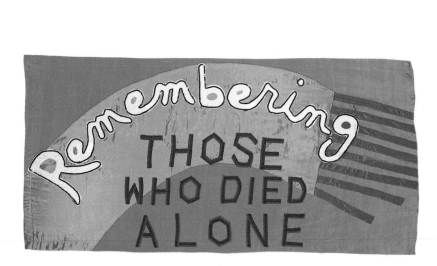

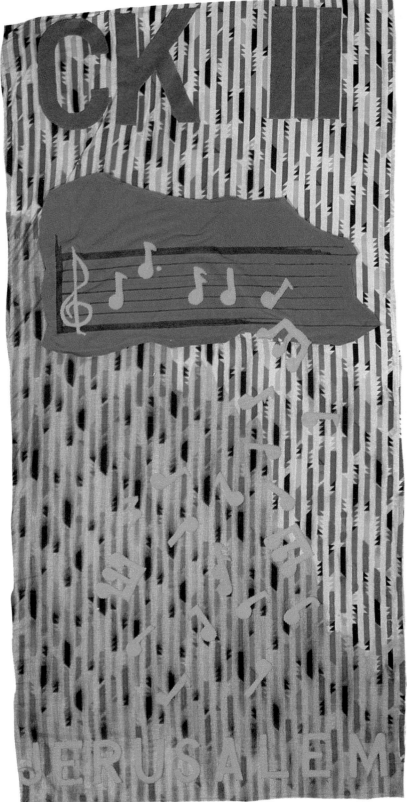

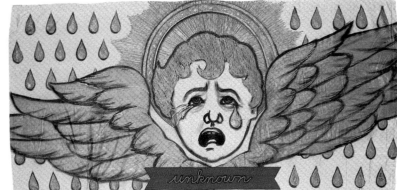

THE BEST DADDY IN THE WORLD
DIED OF AIDS
ON MARCH 2, 1987
I LOVE YOU FOREVER DADDY! ❤, BABYDOLL

Larry L. is my father. He always was so proud of me. He always gave me such confidence in myself. We could talk about everything from friends to movies to genetic engineering. When I was 10, he explained the theory of relativity to me. He always wanted me to learn and question. How I wish he had more time. I still have so many things to learn from him. God, I love him so much! My sorrow is endless.

This project has allowed me to understand what happened a little better.

Thank you,
Diane

Diane, a senior at the University of California at Berkeley, proudly wrote her father's full name on a panel. She couldn't fit the word "love" on the last line, so she painted a red heart in front of the words "baby doll," her father's nickname for her. "I'm really happy with it," says Diane. "It's what I wanted to say — his name, the facts and that I loved him." Diane's mother, however, fearful that people may recognize her husband, asked that his name be blacked out.

Diane wrote to The NAMES Project in April 1987, after seeing a tiny mention in the newspaper of a portable monument for people who died of AIDS. Her father had died a month earlier. "I was really in pain," she said. "But it was something I still could do that wasn't too difficult." Her mother bought the fabric, but Diane worked on the piece alone. "It was my own personal thing," she said. "It really helped me. In many ways, I can't believe that he's gone. Working on this project made it a bit more real. I know that he is not coming back."

Larry L., a gay married man, kept his gay life separate from his daughter. "I had a loving family to go home to," says Diane. "I love him. I always will love him. He was such a wonderful, loving father."

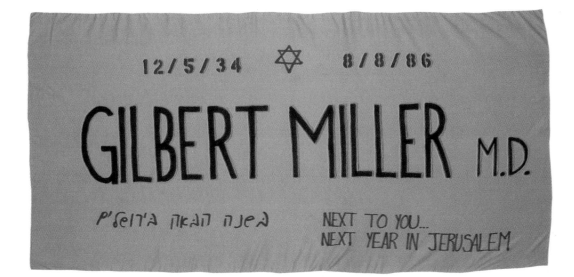

12/5/34 ✡ 8/8/86

GILBERT MILLER M.D.

גבעה הבאה בירושלים

NEXT TO YOU...
NEXT YEAR IN JERUSALEM

June 1986, was a proud month for Dr. Gilbert Miller because both his sons were graduated from college. First he flew from his home in Bayside, Queens, to California State Sacramento, where his eldest son, Seth, received a bachelors degree in Computer Science. One week later, he drove to Ithaca, New York, for Larry's graduation from Cornell. Dr. Miller looked twenty years older than his 51 years, and was wearing a wig, a goatee and makeup. He prayed that the people sitting next to him didn't notice his Kaposi's sarcoma lesions. Immediately after Larry's graduation, he took a two-week vacation to Israel. The two weeks were a graduation present for Larry, but they were also a gift to himself. Gilbert had never been to Israel, and it was important to him that he make the trip before he died.

When he returned from Israel, Gilbert was hospitalized. He had stopped eating and taking his medication. His lungs filled with fluid, and he could no longer speak. He banged on his bed with frustration. On August 8, 1986, Dr. Gilbert Miller died. At his bedside were his ex-wife, his mother-in-law, and two of his three children, all from a marriage that had ended eight years earlier when Gilbert realized he could no longer live a heterosexual life.

Seth was not nearby when his father died. Only two days earlier his parents had convinced him that it would be best that he return to his programming job in California. There, Seth recruited a friend to help him make his father's panel. They ran around Pay 'n Save buying assorted glitters and glues. But when the time came, these were never used. Instead, Seth chose simply to write, in both Hebrew and English, "Next year in Jerusalem."

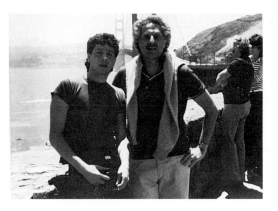

Gilbert Miller with his son Seth.

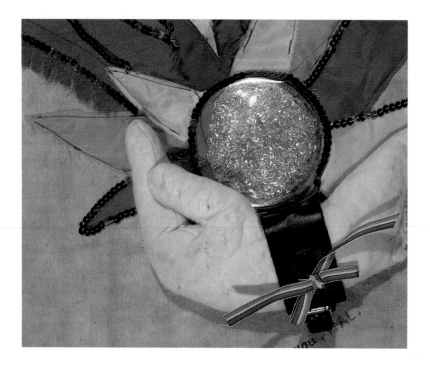

Hal Marret was that ray of sunshine
on a cloudy day.
He was the love in love songs.
A sweet and gentle soul.

And oh what he could make you feel in bed,
and in your head.

Rest well Hal.
I will think of you often.

And Hal,
keep the bed warm.

  Christopher Priestly

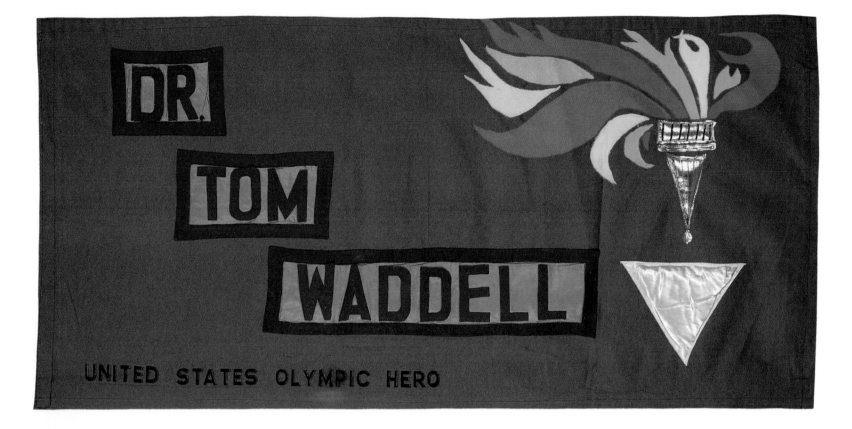

r. Tom Waddell, an Olympic decathlete, founded the Gay "Olympic" Games. Just before Waddell died of AIDS, the Supreme Court ruled in favor of the United States Olympic Committee against Waddell and the Gay Games' use of the word "Olympic."

This is my second quilt. The first quilt for my friend, Hal Marret, was one of the most difficult things I have ever done. When it was completed, it took two weeks before I could turn it loose to become part of The NAMES Project.

Such pain! There are many tears, much grief, and love beyond words in Hal's quilt. Every stitch is a stitch of love.

My quilt for Dr. Tom Waddell was quite the opposite. Dr. Waddell and I met on several occasions, nothing more, nothing less.

This is my quilt, not of love and understanding, but of anger, hurt, and tears. But these tears are "Tears of Rage" (thank you, Bob Dylan) . . . such powerful words . . . TEARS OF RAGE.

Every stitch in Dr. Tom Waddell's quilt is a stitch of rage — for the insensitivity of the present administration to act against this epidemic, for the misunderstanding of some, but most of all to the United States Supreme Court for their denial of the use of the word "Olympic" associated with games Dr. Waddell founded.

Shame on you!!

Shame on you, not only for the denial of the use of the word "Olympic," but also shame on you that my quilt for Dr. Thomas Waddell doesn't have love in every stitch.

What is so incredibly sad to me is that such a thing as The NAMES Project is needed. I do hope that when the next showing is unveiled, my name won't be one of those included. If it is, I would like to express some tears, lots of love and also some anger.

Tears of rage? You bet!

A. Christopher Priestly

Peter Heth was the production designer of **Tokens**, a play on the Great Plague of London in 1665. "The parallels between AIDS and the Plague were undeniable," says **Tokens** performer Christine Haupert. Peter spent over six months designing the award-winning sets for this massive theatrical spectacle. He designed hundreds of "dead body" dummies that were tossed into plague pits throughout the play. Three cast members from this 1985 San Francisco production — Paul Cyr, Christine Haupert and Dan Turner — attached one of these figures, with its arm draped across its face, to Peter's memorial panel.

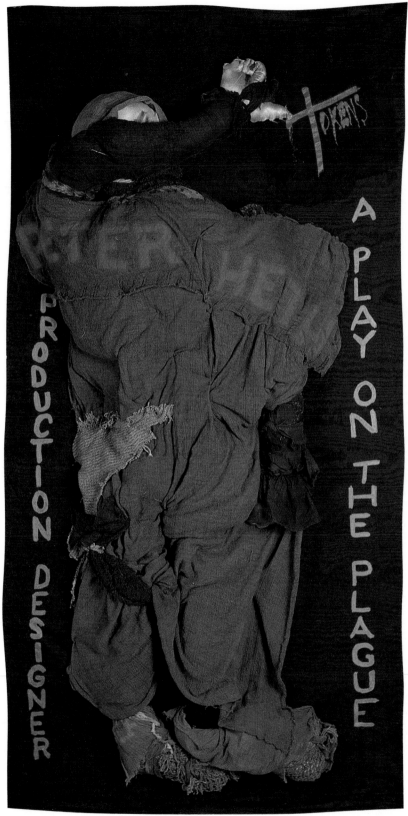

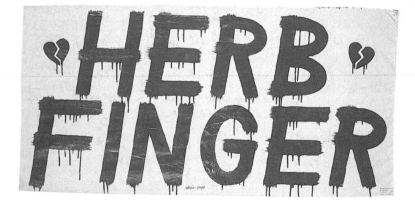

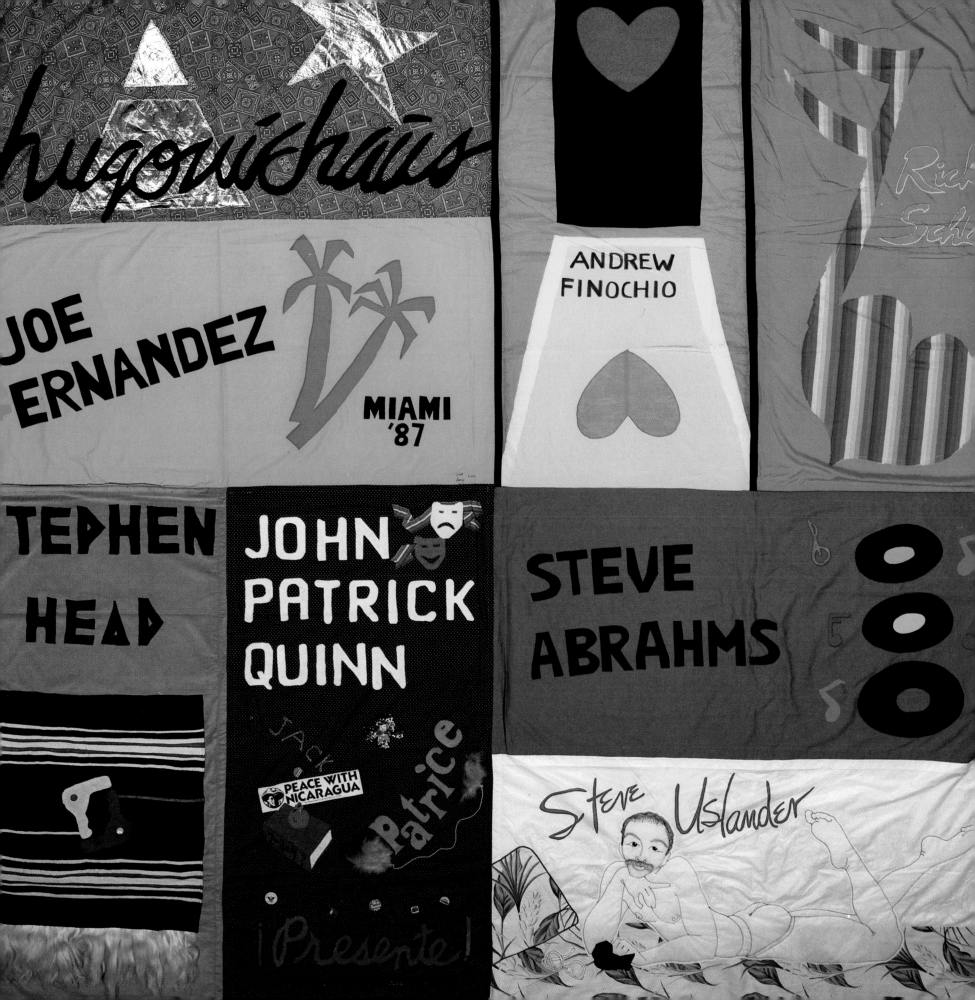

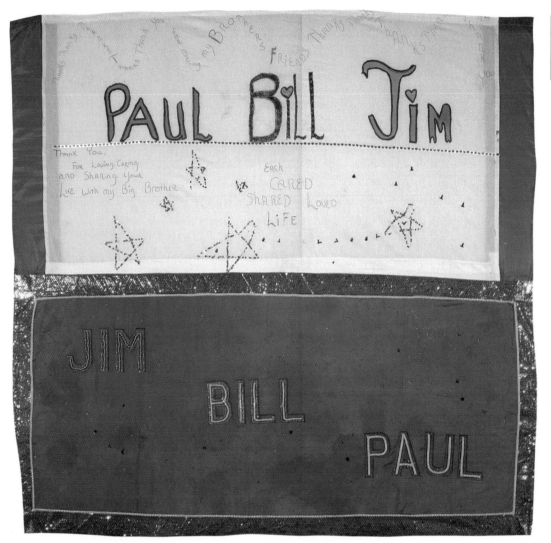

Michael's younger sister, living in Los Angeles, made the panel with the sequined stars. "I made this panel for my Big Brother's family, Jim, Bill and Paul," she writes to The NAMES Project. "They cared a lot about my brother in life and I want them remembered." Karen Webb, a friend of Michael's from Cincinnati, Ohio, made the second panel for the three friends.

Michael, Paul, Jim and Bill did the cosmic sixties together. Parties, drugs and rock 'n' roll, the Age of Aquarius, Maharishi and pilgrimages to Katmandu. They grew their hair, wore Indian headbands, knocked around New York for a while, discovered psychedelics, Janis Joplin and Eastern mysticism. They moved to California, full of West Coast optimism. It was one great hell-raising, consciousness-expanding trip. Often they drifted to different cities, but no matter where they were, they were always together — four best friends on a great twenty-five-year adventure.

Paul Harman and Michael Kensinger met first. They were both 16 in South Bend, Indiana. They'd meet at 2 A.M. at the Greyhound bus station, the local teenage hangout, and dance all night to such jukebox favorites as the Four Seasons's "Big Girls Don't Cry."

One year later, Michael introduced Paul to Jim Calderone, a graduate student in English literature at Notre Dame, whom Michael had met at a Christmas party following a prayer meeting. Michael and Jim discovered that they had lived around the block from each other as infants in Galesburg, Illinois. Jim introduced Paul and Michael to Bill Bell, an undergraduate Jim had met in the Notre Dame Glee Club. This was the beginning of their four-man lifetime friendship.

Paul was the traveler who led the group everywhere. "We pulled off so many trips together," reminisces Michael. "Some great ones, some weird ones. Acid trips through steamy swamps and train trips to the Taj Mahal. VW bus trips across America. Cosmic trips. But the part I liked best was when we would talk and talk and talk, and spin ourselves into ever-expanding talk."

Bill was the avant-garde trend-seeker — always on the cutting edge. He had a massive collection of books and records.

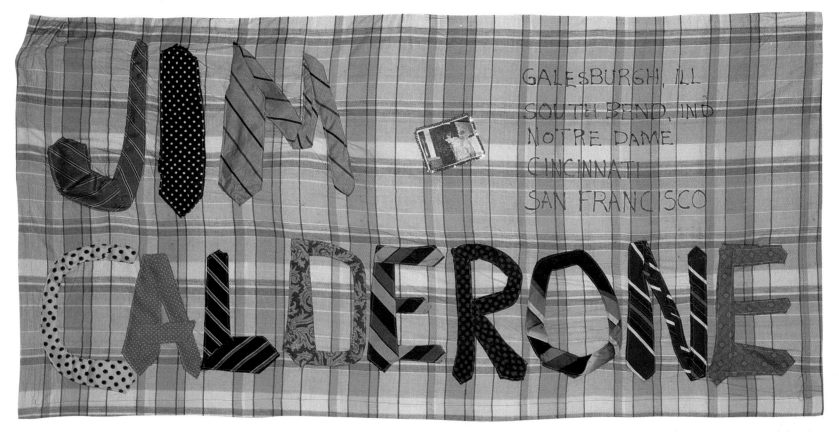

GALESBURGH, ILL
SOUTH BEND, IND
NOTRE DAME
CINCINNATI
SAN FRANCISCO

"The neckties are for Jim the teacher and linguist," says Michael. "They're for his dapper, erudite and straightforward side, and the soft, flannel background is for the gentle, warm, funny friend with the best laugh."

He introduced the guys to Gonzo journalism and Tom Wolfe, the hippest new underground clubs and the hottest new bands. They'd hop planes from wherever they were and meet for rock concerts given by the Rolling Stones, Jefferson Airplane, The Who or Bruce Springsteen.

Michael was the entrepreneur, always involving the four of them in business ventures. In the late seventies, Michael was working as a candle-maker in Cincinnati, Jim was teaching high school and Bill was bartending in Chicago. The three of them packed two trucks and joined Paul, who had settled in San Francisco six years before. There, Michael devised projects for the crew. They opened a candle-mak-

ing store on Pier 39. They invested in real estate, remodeling old Victorian houses. They ran bars. Paul loved cats, so they opened a specialty store on Fisherman's Wharf full of cat paraphernalia, called "Cat mon Dieu."

As Michael remembers it, "We were real typical guys. Nothing special. We were born in the right day and age with a lot of freedom, and we chose to explore it. I see that as special, but it's a pretty normal story of that time, to float around doing stuff."

Then the never-ending party started to falter. Jim began to complain of one mysterious neurological symptom after the next. As early as 1977, while still in

Chicago, Jim kept going to doctors, participating in one medical study after another. When he moved to San Francisco, his friends hoped that a change of scene would make a difference. Jim managed the candle shop, but he'd come to work late. "He'd close the shop early," says Michael. "He just couldn't stay awake." For years, Paul, Bill and Michael tried to figure out what was going on. They thought that Jim was tired because he was bored or unhappy. They just didn't know.

Then Bill started getting sick. It was severe hepatitis. Jim, although he was tired all the time, helped Bill recover. A year later, Jim went back to the hospital — San Francisco General, Ward 5A. There were warning signs taped across his door. The doctors took Paul, Bill and Michael aside and told them about this new disease — AIDS.

In 1983, Jim was still at San Francisco General and Bill was back at Kaiser Hospital, seriously ill. Michael and Paul ran between hospitals, caring for their two dearest friends. By this time, Jim was in dementia. He was blind. He hadn't shaved for days. "When we visited him, they said to put on gloves and gowns and masks," says Michael. "I did. When his mother came to take him home, I shaved him and I helped him put on his pants because he couldn't remember how. I hugged him for the last time. Oh, Jim. Who knew back then? Who knew?" All four friends were never together again.

Even with Jim gone, Michael and Paul had a full-time job taking care of Bill. He'd lost a lot of weight and was in a wheelchair, and they were fighting hard to keep him alive. Bill died in the spring of 1984. Paul and Michael scattered his ashes across the San Francisco Bay on a glorious May afternoon.

Oh, Bill, I miss you. The ups and downs, the rock 'n' roll of it all. The twists and turns of our dreams and our dramas. We stuck it all out together. We grew up and we did what we did together. For 20 years, you made me laugh and brought music into my life. We shared our odyssey and gave each other the strength of our hands and hearts.

Paul and I scattered your ashes to the earth and to the water and to the sky. To set you free and to set us free. To take a trip through outer space and be a rocket man. To say good-bye to you and for you to say hello to Jim. Imagine. Blowin' in the wind. See you later Bill. Just my Bill . . .

Then it was Paul's turn. He started getting strange viruses. He would be laid up in bed for a week or two, barely able to eat. On Valentine's Day 1985, Paul's doctor told him that he had pneumocystis. Michael knew the answer but he still called the AIDS Foundation just to be sure that a pneumocystis diagnosis really meant that Paul had AIDS. The Foundation confirmed his fears. For weeks, Paul moved in and out of the hospital until Michael and Sergio, another close friend, brought him home in a hospital bed, with oxygen canisters and Michelle, a full-time nurse. Paul weighed 85 pounds.

One night, Michael, Sergio and Michelle turned Paul's bath into a ceremony. Paul was ready to die, so his friends decided to give him a fantasy trip to Tibet. They lit hundreds of candles, scented his bathing water and floated rose petals in it. They brought his cats into his bedroom. They rolled him into the position of a sleeping Buddha. "It was like having a wake before he died," says Michael. "We didn't know what to do. But you do the best you can and you make it up as you go along." Paul returned to consciousness for a moment. He smiled. Five days later, he died peacefully in the loving care of his friends.

Michael and Paul had said good-bye to their friends together. Now Michael, 44, the sole survivor, threw a party on a yacht in the San Francisco harbor on Paul's birthday — Halloween night 1985, for their final farewell. Under a full moon, surrounded by Paul's friends, Michael set off firecrackers and served birthday cake as he scattered Paul's ashes. Two years later, Michael planned the quilt he would make to honor the 19-year-old guy in the tangerine sweater who used to dance the nights away at the South Bend bus station. "So long, old friend," said Michael. "I know you'll like the banner."

"I wanted to remember all the wonderful times I had with Bill," says Michael who pasted photographs of Bill on the panel: in Golden Gate Park, at a Rolling Stones concert, with Paul, and dressed in rabbit ears and sunglasses at a party the year the Cincinnati Reds won the World Series. The Japanese fabric was a present from Michael for Bill from Tokyo.

It took three weeks to make Paul's panel. Michael and Sergio dug up the heavy-duty sequined fabric that Paul bought in India. "We knew just what to do with this fabulous fabric that had been around the house for years," says Michael. The two cats in the foreground are funerary figures of ancient Egypt put in the tombs of pharaohs to serve them in the afterlife. The pyramids are for Paul's Egyptian phase and the Himalayas are for his Buddhist phase.

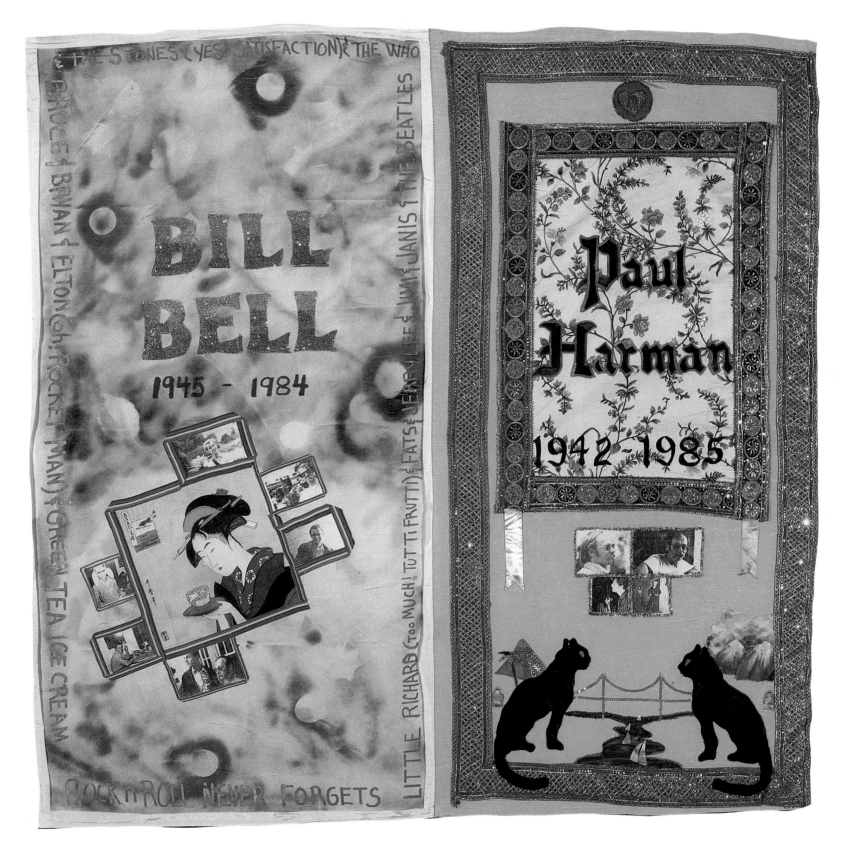

BILL
BELL

1945 – 1984

THE STONES (YES, SATISFACTION) THE WHO

BRUCE & BRYAN & ELTON (oh, ROCKET MAN) & GREEN TEA ICE CREAM

LITTLE RICHARD (TOO MUCH! TUTTI FRUTTI) & FATS & JERRY LEE & JIMI & JANIS & THE BEATLES

ROCK n ROLL NEVER FORGETS

Paul
Harman

1942 – 1985

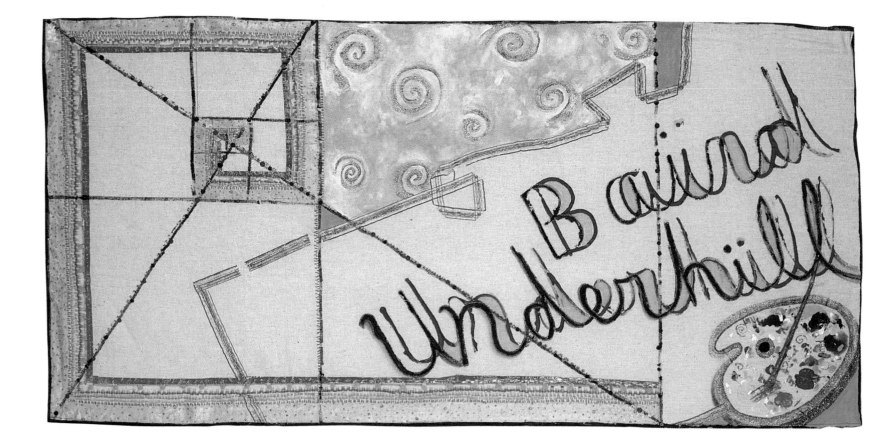

He was lucid and matter-of-fact in telling me that he had gone to
Sirius 2. I said, "The star?" "Yes." "How did you get there?" "By the
starship." He had brought back 200 boxes. In the boxes were amulets
containing a serum — a cure for AIDS. He had already received his
injection on Sirius 2. The boxes were now in his studio in the next room
and he wanted me to look for them. I didn't find them and he responded
with, "Too bad, it must have been a dream."

Later he told me very certainly that the boxes were there. I never
found them and Baird passed away a day later.

His experience, his visit to Sirius 2, was his hope — which I carry
along with mine. The hope for boxes filled with amulets. Ampules filled
with serum. Where they come from doesn't matter. Hoping for them
does.

Steve Newberger
San Francisco

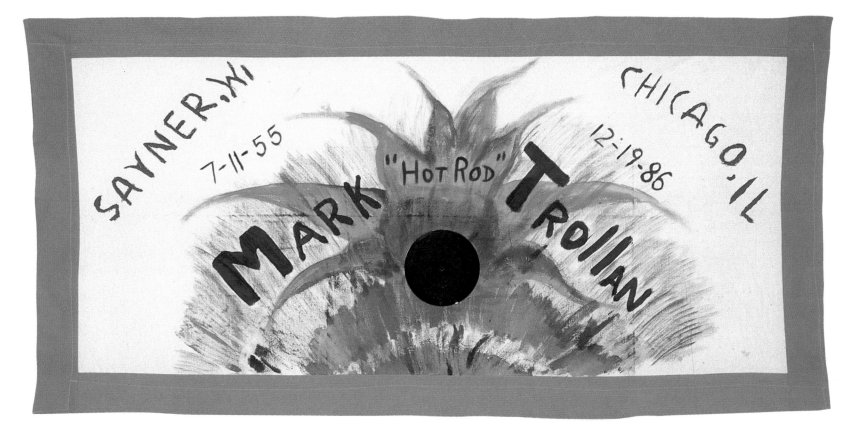

SAYNER.WI 7-11-55

CHICAGO.IL 12-19-86

MARK "HOT ROD" Trollan

I don't quite remember how I met Mark or where, but it seems like it was a long friendship. I do remember that it was business-related. Mark "Hot Rod" Trollan was a deejay and a remix artist, and I owned a local record company. I went to Hot Rod to seek his expertise and one thing led to another and we found out we had a lot more in common than just music.

So we became friends and shared a strong working relationship. And when I myself became sick, going into the hospital, Hot Rod was there with me in the next ward. It worked out well because he was already a pro at all this while I was only just diagnosed.

In the hospital we provided companionship for one another when everyone had gone home. One particular day Hot Rod was very angry about the hopelessness of the doctors. He was preparing for his death. He wanted to talk to his boyfriend. What he wanted to say was, "It's O.K. for you to go out with other men after I die," but it hurt so much. I am glad and proud that I could be there for him.

One day I had to decide whether or not to let them do a particular test. Hot Rod, having had every test in the book, took me aside and told me it would be a piece of cake and not to worry. As soon as the test was over Hot Rod showed up with a piece of cake.

When Hot Rod passed away, his ashes were scattered across the floor of his favorite club. And so went Mark "Hot Rod" Trollan.

My Friend!

ver since he managed a high school rock band at 13, David Bell dedicated his life to the music business. For 17 years, he worked as a backstage manager and toured with such well-known performers as Chick Corea and Ted Nugent. Meanwhile, he started his own record label, Persona Records.

But in January 1987, one month after the death of his friend, Mark "Hot Rod" Trollan, David's priorities changed. Since then, he has not bought a single record, and he no longer owns the company he created. He doesn't even listen to the radio anymore. "I switched gears," says David, who was diagnosed with AIDS just before he gave up music. "Now I'm lobbying for people with AIDS."

David does not wish that his life were any different. "Yes, I want to live. Yes, I want it all secure. But don't feel sorry for me," he says. "To fight for your life is a very difficult fight, but I have gained so much. I've learned how to give and to take. I used to be shy and quiet, but now I can't afford to be quiet." Now David makes headlines. In August 1987, he chained himself to the fence of Illinois Governor James Thompson's home to protest a bill calling for mandatory AIDS contact tracing. He has also found the energy and time to make quilt panels for four friends, including Trollan, who died of AIDS. AIDS provoked the once apolitical David to become one of Chicago's most outspoken gay activists. "People aren't just *dying* with AIDS," he says. "People are *living* with AIDS. We need better care, and we can't let them quarantine us."

The day David was told that he had ARC, he packed up his apartment on Chicago's North Side and moved back home with his parents. Six months later, his lover John Tudor also moved into the Bell family home in Niles, an upper-middle-class suburb of Chicago where David grew up. David describes himself as a nice little Jewish boy from the suburbs who went to high school in Skokie, Illinois. "Whatever battles you go through, you are still our son," David's father assures his only child.

David now suffers from Kaposi's sarcoma. His doctors took him off the experimental drug AZT when his white blood count dropped too low. So David tries other ways to help boost his immunity system — Chinese herbs, vitamins, visualization, pentamidine mist therapy, massage therapy, acupuncture, and drugs from Mexico and Israel. "The cards are already laid on the table as far as my life is concerned," David says. "There will be one less person here, but I will have done something for the people who come after me."

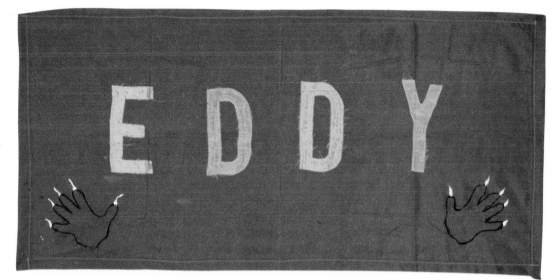

When I was put in the hospital with AIDS, there was an empty bed next to me when I went to sleep. When I woke, Eddy was in the next bed. A slight-built, sickly boy, with fingernails that extended a good inch out and not too clean. He told me that they had said he had AIDS, but he did not understand what that meant and I tried my best to explain and console.

Throughout the next couple of days, I became both his wet nurse and interpreter and friend. You see, AIDS dementia had set in and the doctors and nurses had little time or patience for him. So I was there and Eddy thanked me again and again. I was only glad to have a way to remember him with his panel.

Love, Dave

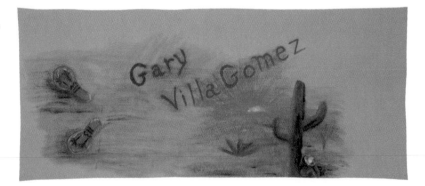

David met little Gary soon after he was diagnosed at an ARC support group meeting. "He was very angry," David remembers. "And he fought his diagnosis to the end."

The last time a mutual friend saw Gary, he was in the hospital, tied to a chair and slumped over. Says David, "He died alone, very scared and very sad."

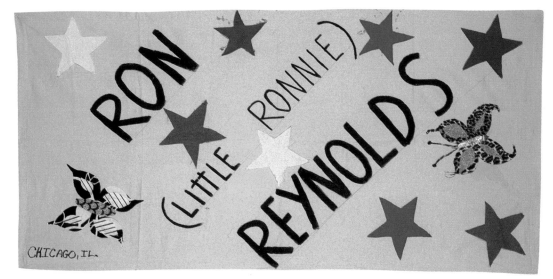

"Little Ronnie" Reynolds and Brian O'Sullivan became friends when they lived in the same Chicago rooming house. They used to play chess for hours. Sometimes Brian would help Ronnie find used parts for his old car, or he'd play with Ronnie's three-year-old son.

Brian never had a close friend with AIDS until Ronnie contracted the disease. After Ronnie died at 21 in December 1986, Brian labored diligently over a quilt panel bearing Little Ronnie's name. Shortly after he finished the job, Brian, 21, also died of AIDS. Brian's name now appears on another panel made by his friend David Bell.

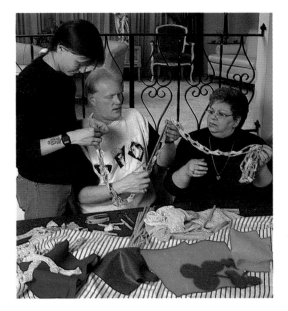

At a sewing bee in his parents' living room, David Bell (center) makes a panel for his friend, 21-year-old Brian O'Sullivan. Dave and Brian met at a drop-in center for people living with AIDS. David's mother and his lover, John Tudor, help add the finishing touches.

Billy Donald worked for the federal government for 30 years. He was appointed by Governor Wallace of Alabama to serve on President Reagan's presidential committee for the handicapped.

Billy Denver Donald was my brother. He was born in Dorsey, Michigan, on June 18, 1936. He died April 23, 1987.

He was a father to a 19-year-old son, a brother to three sisters and son to a widowed mother, and special nephew to many aunts and uncles, a cousin to about 60, a friend, a highly respected manager to his fellow workers and so much more.

I was sitting in the hospital waiting room after just being told Bill had AIDS. I mentally became very small — lifted off the sofa — went out the window and landed on the grass. The wind blew a leaf over me and I hid from the world for a few seconds. With God's help and Bill's courage, we dealt with his illness with all the love within us and life goes on without him. We will miss him forever.

Sincerely,
Norma Shumpert

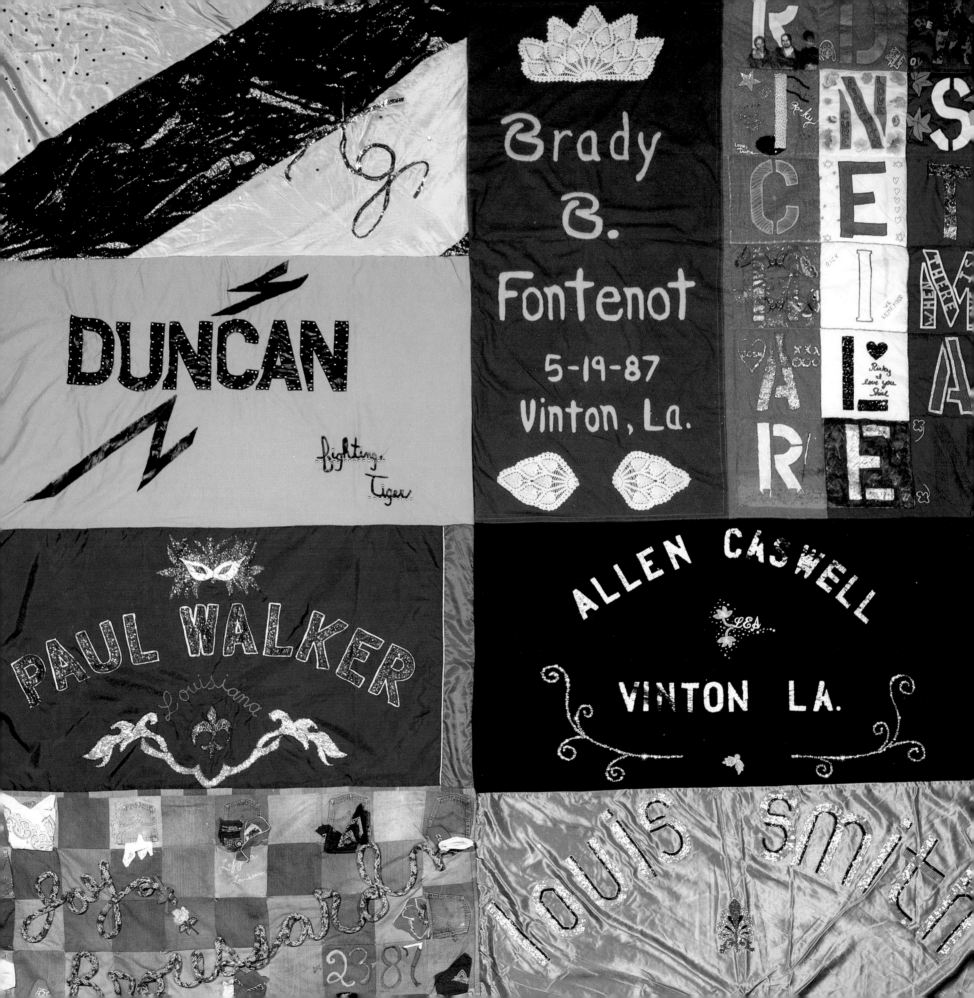

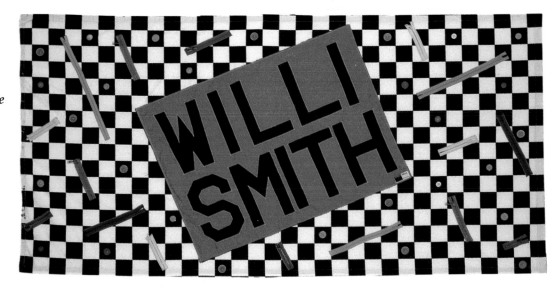

"I really love the way the zippers rattle when you move the panel," says Rod Shelnutt, of the kinetic memorial he made for designer Willi Smith. Shelnutt works all night as a telephone operator and then works as the daytime floor manager at The NAMES Project workshop. "I made this for Willi Smith not just because he was a celebrity, but because he had a real effect on my life."

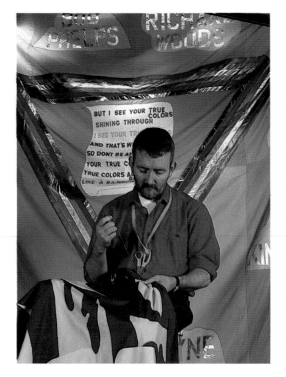

hen sewing enthusiast Rod Shelnutt read the "Volunteers Wanted to Sew" sign in The NAMES Project window, he knew that was the place for him. A self-acclaimed "fabric-aholic," Shelnutt jokes that the reason he moved to San Francisco was to be near Britex, a renowned fabric store. "It's fabric heaven," he laughs in his Georgian drawl.

Rod started sewing at 11 when he made his six-year-old sister a little three-piece outfit all by hand. The pink backless sundress, with bloomers and bonnet to match, so impressed his grandmother that she taught him to use a sewing machine. It has been 24 years of nonstop sewing ever since.

The first really good patterns for men's clothes that Rod was able to find were those designed for Butterick by Willi Smith, a leading New York apparel designer and one of the nation's foremost black entrepreneurs. Indeed, the first clothes Rod ever made for himself were Willi Smith creations.

Rod was shocked when he heard that Willi Smith had died. "I had a flash — an inspiration — a picture of Willi Smith's panel in my head," recalls Rod. "I thought of his designs and colors. He was a very colorful person, so it had to be pure graphic colors." As a final touch to his panel, an explosion of neon zippers and buttons, Rod cut Smith's label off a worn-out tank top, and stitched it to the panel, directly under Smith's name.

Rod was drawn to The NAMES Project for more compelling reasons than his love of fabric. Fourteen of his friends have died of AIDS. He sewed eight vertical panels together, with eight of his friends' names, appliquéd in gold lamé on white clouds, arranged around a rainbow triangle along with the chorus to Cyndi Lauper's hit, "True Colors."

He used six different colors of lamé for the rainbow. "It's my fifty-nine dollar rainbow," Rod says with a smile. "All these people — my friends — weren't ashamed that they had AIDS. They didn't hide the fact they were sick." In order to create this entire 12-by-12-foot quilt with his friends' names, Rod moved everything out of his kitchen and spread the fabric from wall to wall.

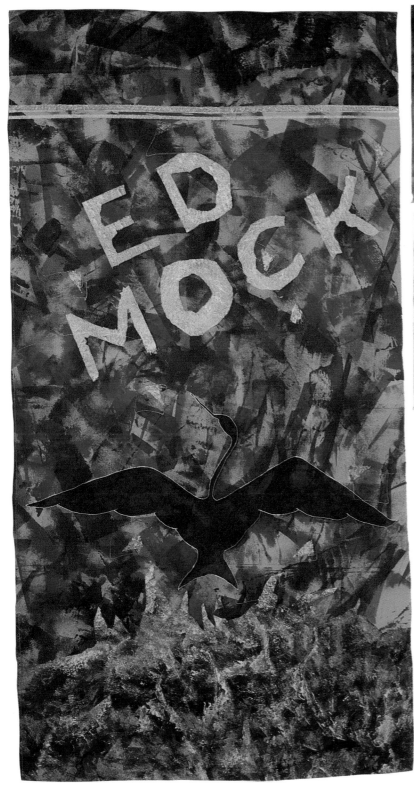

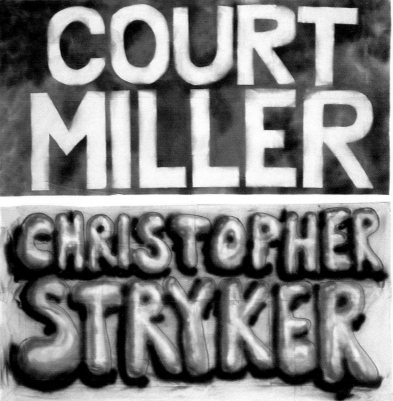

The national arts scene has been devastated by AIDS. Among the hundreds of artists represented in The Quilt are modern-jazz choreographer Ed Mock, filmmaker Arthur J. Bressan Jr., director-choreographer Michael Bennett, avant-garde musician Klaus Nomi, film star Rock Hudson, pianist-entertainer Liberace, actor-pianist Stephen Stucker, New York City Opera singer and director David Hicks, Bay Area opera director Arthur Conrad, performance artist Lari Shox, and guitarist-songwriter Ricky Wilson of the Georgia-based rock group, the B-52's.

Playwright-actor Harvey Fierstein created panels in memory of actors Court Miller and Christopher Stryker who performed with him in his award-winning **Torch Song Trilogy**. Harvey buried Christopher's ashes in the exact same spot in his garden where he painted these cloth memorials.

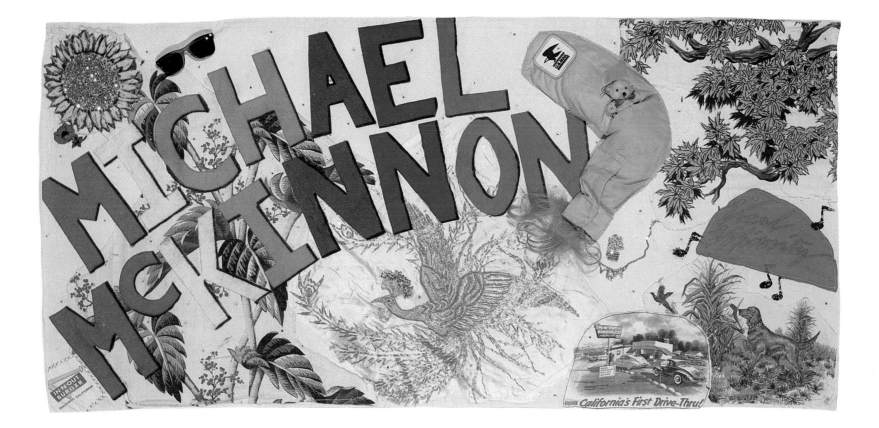

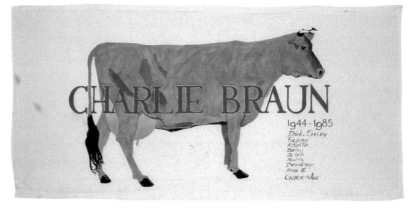

Charlie Braun, psychology professor at U.C. Santa Cruz for seven years, spent most of his adult life living on his 42-acre ranch in Boulder Creek, California. "He loved nature, solitude and the gentleness of cows," writes his friend Dick Oberchain.

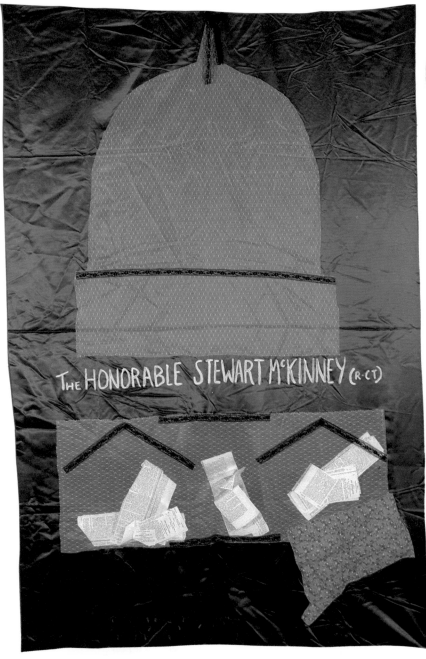

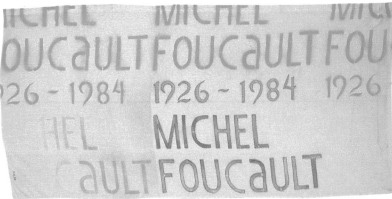

Michel Foucault, a celebrated French intellectual, wrote provocative books on madness, crime, illness and a planned six-volume study on the history of sexuality, which he was half-way through when he died in June 1984. Historian Gerard Koskovich from Stanford, California, interviewed three of Foucault's close friends in Paris in 1985 and wrote the first article in the U.S. that explicitly states that Foucault died of AIDS. Gerard stenciled the philosopher's name in spraypaint in a style typical of the graffiti scrawled all over the walls and sidewalks of the Left Bank.

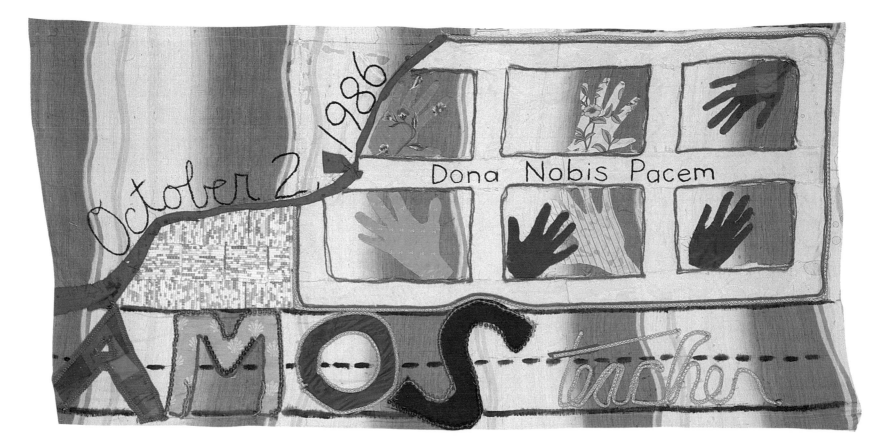

October 2, 1986

Dona Nobis Pacem

AMOS *teacher*

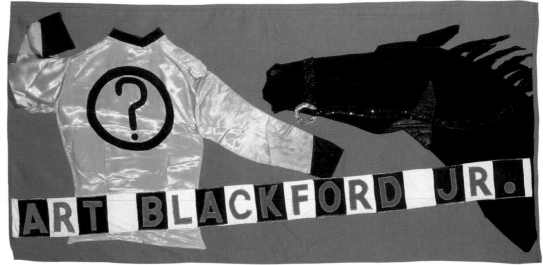

Jim Sherman was 14 when he met the 25-year-old jockey Art Blackford who immediately became his mentor. They bought their first horse together in 1960—a black horse called Denny Did—and worked together for the next 12 years. The racing silks on the panel belonged to Art and were designed by Jim, many years before either of them came out as gay men. "We were intimate but we didn't talk about it," says Jim, now able to understand the significance of the logo he designed when he was 14 years old.

ART BLACKFORD JR.

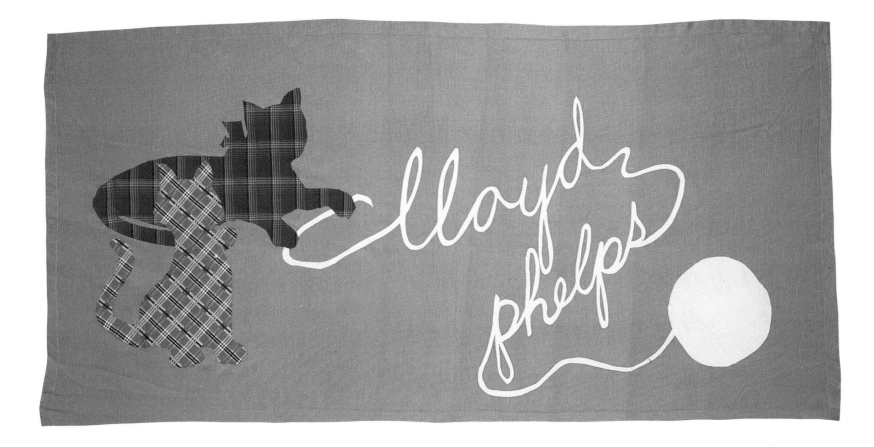

The entire Display Department from Neiman-Marcus's San Francisco store worked on this quilt panel to honor their coworker, Lloyd Phelps. Always dressed in camel-colored trousers and plaid shirts, Lloyd was best know for his creative china, glass and linen displays. His panel, along with 40 others, was featured in the window of San Francisco's Neiman-Marcus store in August 1987.

Lloyd Phelps — an Illinois farm boy with a talent for producing the most elegant and sophisticated table settings. He loved his cats and working on his Victorian flat. He was the gentlest of men, with an improbable deep voice. He was kind, giving and talented, and all of us who worked with him miss him very much.

Neiman-Marcus Visual Presentation Department

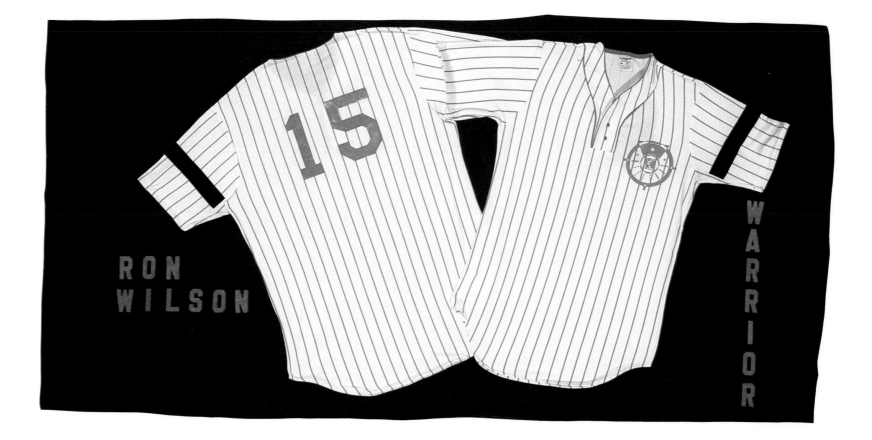

The 1986 Weekend Warrior Softball Team, part of the Hotlanta Softball League, a gay softball group in Atlanta, created this panel for second baseman Ron Wilson. "We wore a black armband on the left arm of our uniforms in memory of people who had died of AIDS," remembers Billy, the shortstop on the team. "We did not know that in a few short months one of our own would fall victim."

I'm lucky that I had a chance to know Ron, but I feel especially sad that I only knew him as a softball player. I'm not sure that we had that much in common other than softball, yet I find myself thinking about him at the craziest times. Maybe I think of him so often because he was the first person I knew who had been taken away with AIDS or maybe it's because he was taken so quickly and so violently or maybe it's so unfair that "only the good die young."

Ron showed tremendous courage during his battle with AIDS. You see, while the rest of us were called warriors, Ron was a Warrior.

Teammate Billy L.

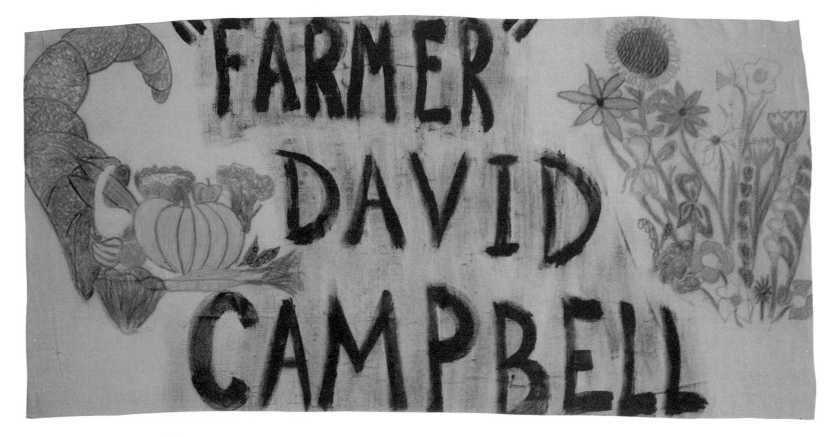

illy King, a potter from Eureka Springs, Arkansas, painted this panel in honor of David Campbell, his former lover. They hadn't seen each other in three years.

Dear David,

I remember the garden dinners we'd prepare, particularly Thanksgiving. And warming our toes on the hearth before going off to bed and making love under the heavy comforter. I'd awaken to the smell of a large farm breakfast, and you'd be off again to your ever-expanding gardens.

I got involved in other things and other people, and we had our parting. I went east and you went west. A friend showed me a letter you had written saying you were sick. Also that I had been the love of your life. We'd never shared these words.

Your spirit lives on in the land you so loved.

With love and fond memories, Billy

107

erry Holcomb ranked at the top of his profession as a costume designer and dresser. He created outfits for the San Francisco Opera, the San Francisco Ballet, and such films as *The Ewok, Howard the Duck* and *Wildfire*. He was the principal dresser on tour with *Dreamgirls*. Jerry was also a landscape architect, who redesigned the gardens at the landmark Mendocino Hotel, and was a past president of the American Fuchsia Society. His hobby was decorating Fabergé-style jeweled eggs.

Jim Ponder, a costumer at the American Conservatory Theater in San Francisco, incorporated pink lamé and chiffon rosebuds into his panel honoring Jerry. These fabrics resemble those of *La Cage aux Folles*, the last play Jerry outfitted. Jerry and Jim worked together for many years at the San Francisco Opera. Jerry was very private about his four-year struggle with ARC, and only in the last few months did his colleagues begin to link his frequent illnesses to AIDS.

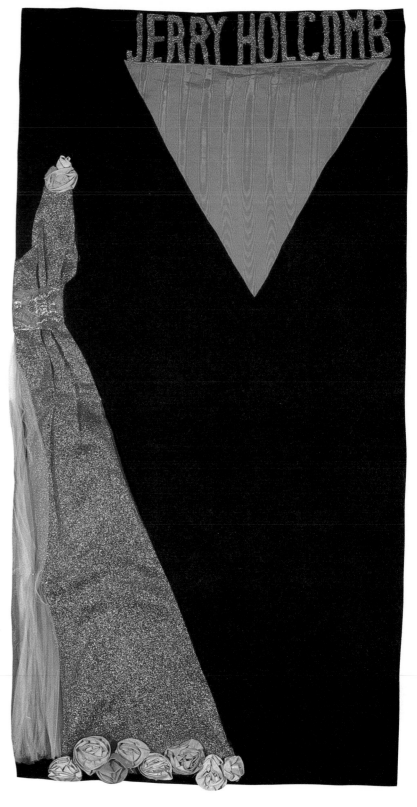

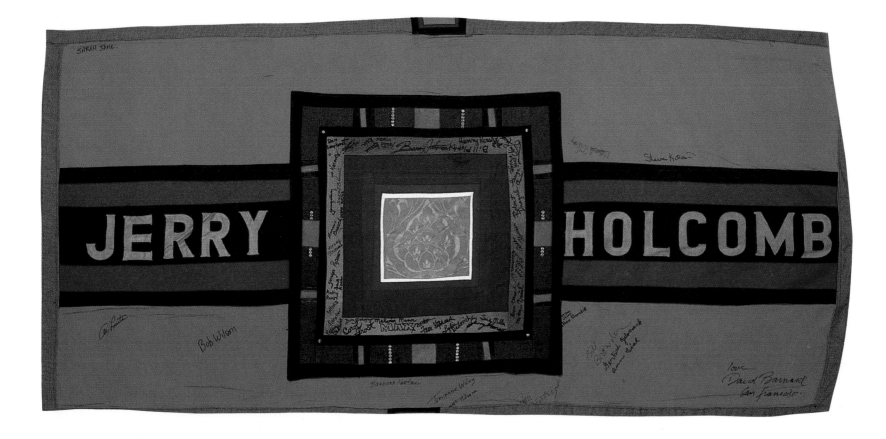

David Barnard sewed with Jerry for 20 years. Together they dyed tights, repaired curtains, made costumes, and stitched bags, tents and seat covers. They perfected a spandex boot to fit over ballet shoes for dance productions of *The Tempest* and *Stars and Stripes*.

David sewed into his panel a piece of gold fabric from the Old Grand Drape at the San Francisco Opera House. Jerry and David mended this curtain often while working for the opera and ballet. When the curtain wore out completely, they cut it up and sold the pieces. The rhinestones are from his tour with *Dreamgirls* and his jeweled eggs. The denim was snipped from Jerry's blue jeans. David cut out a piece of a cape for the peacock-blue background to represent a peacock costume

Jerry designed for Halloween. The maroon silk comes from the lining of a leather bag Jerry made for David. Seventy-five of Jerry's friends, colleagues and fellow members of the theatrical wardrobe union signed the panel. Jerry's lover of 20 years, Barry Jalonack, along with two other friends, helped David with the panel. Immediately after Jerry's memorial service, the four of them delivered their cloth remembrance to The NAMES Project.

Jerry and David put pockets on everything. For Jerry's pickup truck, they designed Levi's seat covers with extra pockets sewn around the sides to hold change, coffee cups and tools. For the "man that doesn't want to take his boots off," they designed "bachelor quilts," durable, denim coverings full of pockets

for the *TV Guide*, cigarettes and any odds and ends around the bed.

On the back of Jerry's panel, David stitched a Levi's pocket. He found the black leather pocket flap with red piping on Jerry's worktable. Inside, David tucked a letter describing the significance of each swatch of fabric used in the panel.

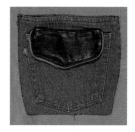

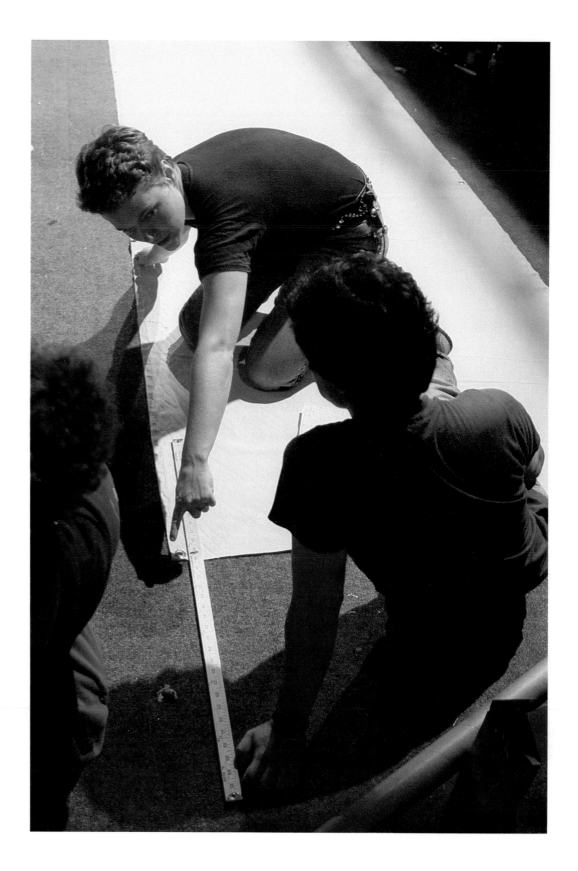

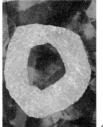

ctober 4, 1987 — one week before The Quilt's inaugural display in Washington.

Last week, The NAMES Project headquarters served as a creative center to decorate panels. Now, as October 11 approaches, it has become an all-night sweatshop where volunteers put in countless hours piecing individual quilt panels together, grommeting 2,000 yards of white walkway material, and packing The Quilt up for its trip to Washington.

The excitement of the final week draws the crew even closer together. One volunteer pins, another hems, and a third sews the eight panels together to form a 12-by-12-foot square. Then each square is bordered with white canvas and handed over to the grommeting team. Once grommeted, the square is labeled and stacked in a storeroom at the back of the workshop, which is filled to capacity already. By the September 15 deadline, the Project had received a total of 800 panels, but in the last four days another 1,200 panels arrived. Dan Carmell can't log them into the computer fast enough.

It's a sweltering Sunday, over 100 degrees, and all three fans are directed at the freshly painted, 50-foot-long signature sash, emblazoned with The NAMES Project logo, which is draped over the balcony to dry. The white fabric for the nine-foot-wide walkways, which will form the gridwork of The Quilt, is everywhere.

Ron Cordova is tense. Cleve Jones is the Project's spokesman, Mike Smith must find the money, but it is Ron who will make The Quilt actually happen. "If one grommet is off," he worries, "if anything was measured incorrectly, there's a chance of losing it all."

Steve Abeyta made elaborate charts to line up the metal eyelets — the grommets. "Now this is man's work," says grommeter Neil Smith, waving a hammer as he teases the men on the sewing machines. Rod Shelnutt, Dan Carmell, Neil Smith and John Wilson became the grommeting team of the final hour. Dan measured, John cut holes in the material with a razor blade, Rod stuck the metal grommets in, and Neil walked behind, hammering. "Grommeting is like doing deep knee bends for five hours," moans Rod Shelnutt. "I can hardly stand up." At 7 P.M., Dan hands the hammer to Ron and the crowd cheers as Ron pounds in the last metal ring.

After dinner, Ron clears out the workshop completely, shoving sewing machines against the walls. As he lays out four 12-by-12-

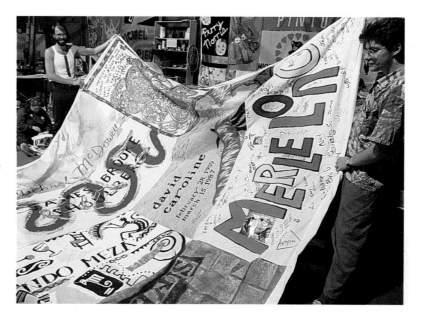

foot squares on the ground, all names facing out so that they can be read from any direction, volunteers fasten them together with plastic cable ties. These 24-by-24-foot blocks will be the real squares of the giant quilt.

The final folding as they prepare to pack the quilts into the plane is a formal event. Each quilt panel is treated with reverence. The volunteers have removed their shoes and step gingerly around The Quilt. "You're laying people's possessions — parts of people — on the ground," Ron tells his emotional crew, "but you can't be afraid of The Quilt. In order to fold it up, you *have* to walk on it."

There are eight folders — just as there will be eight unfolders in the Washington ceremony. "Corners! Fold! Clippers!" Ron bellows as four folders walk their corners to the center, the quilt billowing around them. Spectators lean over the second-floor railing and the front windows are lined all night as passersby watch in awe. The folding teams grow progressively high-spirited. With arms extended in grand arabesques and singing "Come Together Right Now," they hop toward the center of the quilt square in unison. Scott Lago, his mouth full of plastic ties, stops the ceremony for a minute to admire the handiwork on the reverse side of an embroidered panel. By 2 A.M., everyone is exhausted, laughing and hugging. Ten members of the Gay Men's Chorus stop in to sing an Irish blessing of good-bye, good traveling and good luck. People leave reluctantly. There is a sadness that it is over — for the time being.

At 9 o'clock the following morning, the U-Haul truck arrives. It's the hottest day on record in San Francisco. In pairs, volunteers carefully carry the ordered 24-by-24-foot squares to the truck. They line the bottom of the U-Haul with the walkway material and pack The Quilt so that the panels are sandwiched between border sashes. The U-Haul pulls away, and there is an eerie empty feeling left in the workshop now that The Quilt has gone.

The Flying Tigers, the world's largest cargo carrier, will fly The Quilt to Washington and back. Seventy employees donated money or benefits to the safe journey of The Quilt. Flight attendant Jeff Kuball arranged the entire trip. Jeff drives the U-Haul to the airport loading area, and together with Ron, Scott, Jack and Eve, he watches The Quilt being carried by two forklifts to be weighed. When the scale reads 6,890 pounds, Jeff's jaw drops. It is over double the average DC-10 container weight. Ron, who has been lifting The Quilt all week, isn't surprised. "Ten thousand grommets . . . 70,000 feet of seams . . . 2,000 yards of walkway material . . . 1,920 names . . . so much love, so much loss . . . my dear friend Drew," Ron muses as he watches The Quilt move along the conveyer belt bound for Washington, D.C.

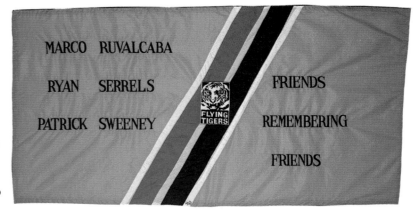

Flying Tigers, the air freight company that transported The Quilt to Washington, made a banner for three of their crew out of fabric from around the world. While in Anchorage, flight attendant Jeff Kuball, who designed the panel to resemble the Tiger planes, roller-skated four miles to pick up the blue, red and white material. The Tiger logo came off a garment bag made in the Okinawa Islands and the sewing was done in Seoul, South Korea, by the tailor who usually embroiders personnel names on flight bags.

ROBERT "SCOTTY" SCOTT

WM. "BILL" CONNERS

CHARD DONOVAN

PAUL "MARILYN"

DENNIS RYAN

ROB FRYE

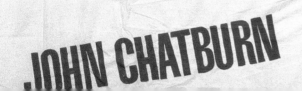

JOHN CHATBURN

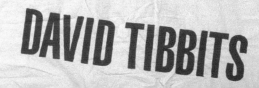

DAVID TIBBITS

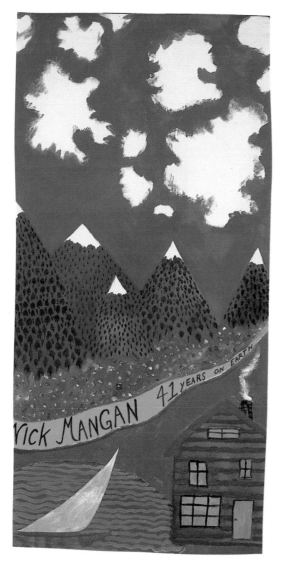

urrounded by cans of paint and brushes on a living room floor, two men on their hands and knees planned a memorial for Nick Mangan. Both needed to make a statement about AIDS. Jerry Mangan wanted the commemorative panel to express his own sorrow, or perhaps even anger about his brother's death from AIDS. Rollie Kennedy, who never met Nick but knew about him through Jerry, needed to create a public memorial to the life of another gay man. "As a gay man sharing in the grief of a straight man's loss, I was honored to work on this panel," says Rollie.

After staring at the blank canvas for a while, not knowing where to start, Jerry and Rollie began painting the blue sky. Nick always wanted to settle back in Colorado, where the three Mangan brothers grew up. "When I think of Colorado, it's the sky that I think of first," says Jerry, "lots and lots of fluffy clouds." Slowly, Rollie and Jerry worked down the canvas, never quite sure what they were going to do next.

As they splattered paint, they talked less about Nick, and more about the way they lived their own lives in Province-town, Massachusetts, trying to make it as adults. Until Nick became ill, Jerry and Rollie knew each other only well enough to stop and chat on the street, but had little in common. In June 1987, Jerry, a sculptor and a counselor for adult schizo-phrenics, left for the family home in Greeley, Colorado, to help his 76-year-old mother take care of Nick. While he was in Colorado, Jerry received understanding, tender letters from Rollie, who was moved by word of Nick's illness. "He touched me deeper than anyone," says Jerry. "This ill-ness is a real deadly thing, but it does bring people together."

Nick Mangan was my younger brother. It saddened me to say we never knew each other well. When we were able to meet in those rare instances as adults, it was all too obvious he and I belonged to separate worlds. We both understood that we wanted a connection with each other, but we just couldn't seem to find the path.

There were times that Nick and Jerry didn't see one another for five-year periods. Even when Nick, a businessman and chemical engineer, became ill, he and Jerry were not very close. Their lives were too different. But when Jerry left his job, girlfriend and 10-year-old daughter behind to care for his brother, everything changed. "It was at that point I began to know my little brother again," he says. "With our different values and our differ-ent sexual life-styles, we didn't have all that much to talk about. But we did care about each other. I knew that I had to be with him."

When Jerry arrived in Colorado, he wanted to talk to his brother about dying, metaphysics, alternative medicine and health foods. This was not Nick's style. Instead, they expressed their closeness each time Jerry would carry Nick to the bathroom, or whenever he rubbed vitamin E oil over the KS lesions on Nick's face, or the times Jerry climbed into the bath with Nick to help lower him into the tub. "We laughed, we grew silent, we cursed the dis-ease, we believed in miracles, and I read to him of dying as he slept," says Jerry.

Jerry vividly remembers all the times when Nick would get out of bed and try to stand up, forgetting that he couldn't walk. "It was very tough for his pride to allow me to pick him up," says Jerry. "It is intimacy with a capital 'I' — the intimacy of being close to someone when they are really in need, and staying — not running.

"My mom and I went through a lot together," Jerry says. "Sometimes I think we felt like people who have gone through a war."

Dear Mark,

   I'd rather have you alive and sick than dead and gone, but I know you suffered. Through it all I knew that you didn't want to have to die and you told me you'd really miss this earth. Well, this earth certainly misses you, toots! I miss calling you for late night chats and eating with you. I miss hearing you bitch about school, but most of all I miss holding you tight and lying with you as we slept. I miss looking directly into your eyes, which by the by I could not close when you died. Mark, I will go to my grave thinking of you.

   Much love, John

P.S. Write back if you can.

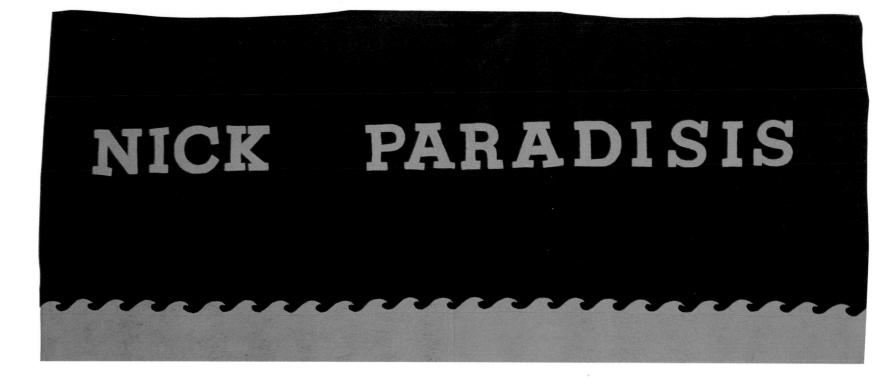

NICK PARADISIS

ick Paradisis, 39, adored his live-in lover Jane and his three big dogs. As a healthy, muscular athlete, he loved to water-ski and, even when he became ill, Nick continued to spend weekends skiing at the Berkeley Marina until he became too weak. Just before Nick died, Jane, 36, who had been with him constantly through his illness, called her friend Marty and Reverend Janie Spahr to visit their Marin County home.

We came and sat with Nick and talked with him. We began talking about the Light and going to the Light. Marty told Nick he would walk with Jane and the dogs on the beach that Nick loved, that Jane would be O.K., that he could go. When Marty said that, Nick's pulse and breathing slowed way down. Jane knew that Nick was dying. He was letting go. His eyes focused as Marty said, "Go to the Light, Nick. Greet your friends . . . " and we felt him leave us. Jane saw peace on his face. His eyes were beautiful and the lesions on his face disappeared. Nick, who fought so hard to live, died with such peace. His face was free of all the pain — something Jane needed to see. At last there was peace.

Reverently submitted, Janie Spahr

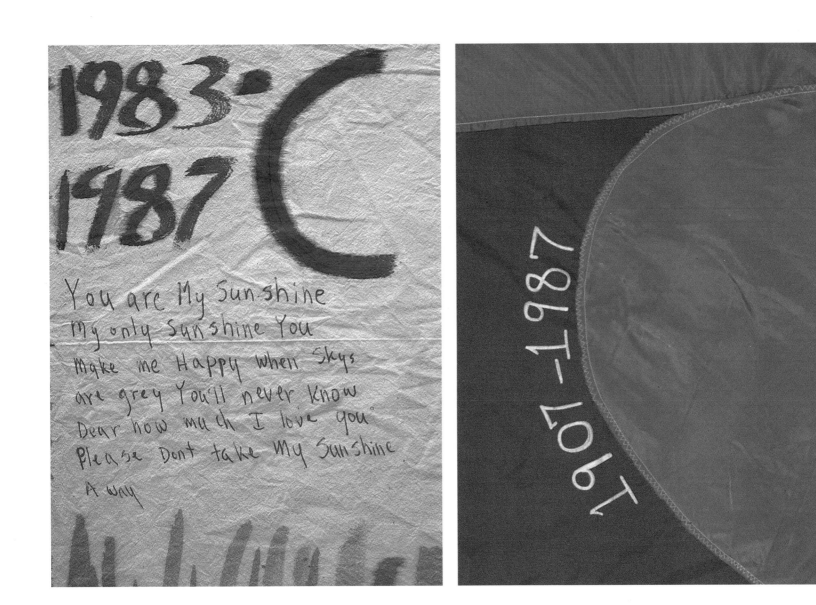

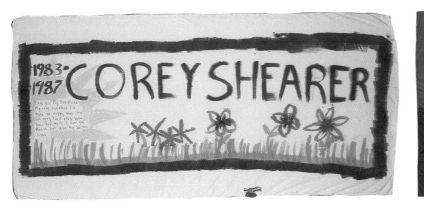

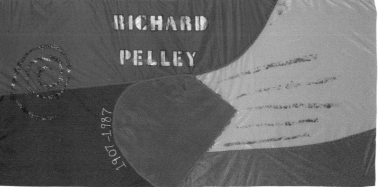

117

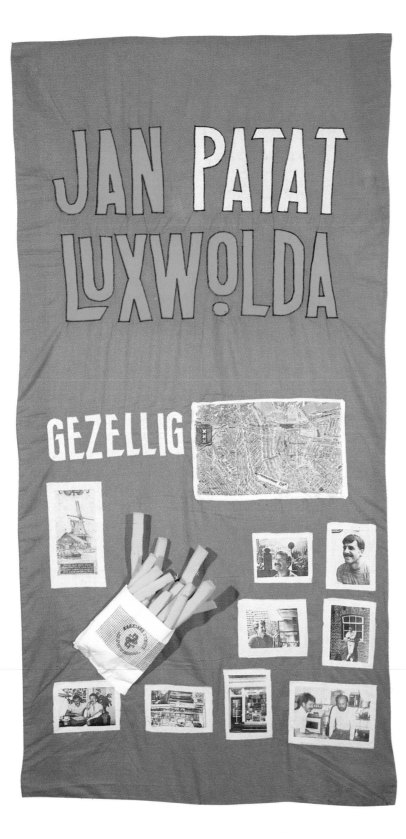

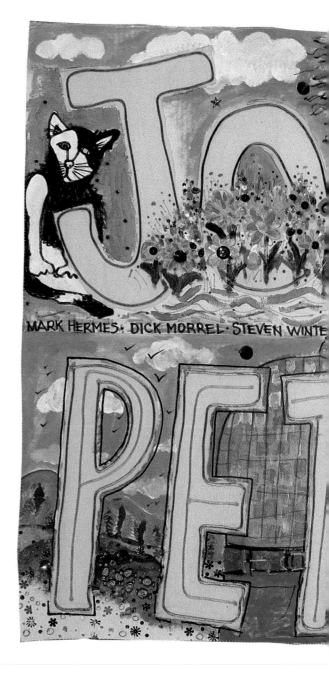

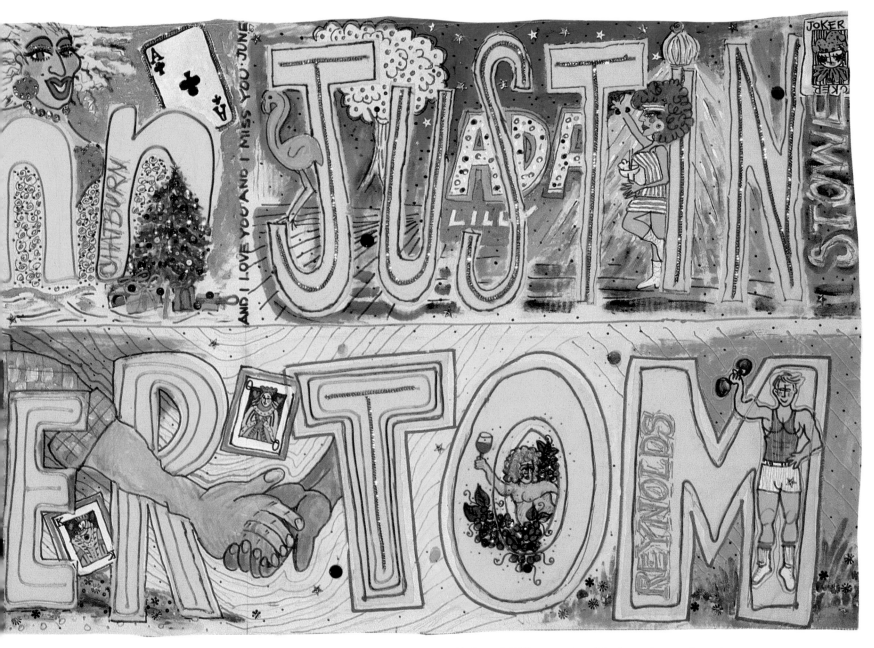

Robert Millington lost his four closest friends in one year. He first met John Chatburn, Justin Stone, Peter Hogg and Tom Reynolds in San Francisco in 1968 when they became roommates. They loved drag, and regularly won prizes for their Halloween costumes. Robert drew Peter and Tommy, lovers for 11 years, holding hands. The day after Tommy's death, Peter went into dementia and he died six weeks later. The names in small print on the panel are other friends of Robert who have died of AIDS. Robert remembers John and Justin's last words to him: "Keep on. Don't let this stop you, too."

Aaron John Miller loved to sew. By sixth grade, he was creating original designs on his mother's sewing machine at the family ranch in Florence, Arizona. In the sixties, the Miller family opened a local chain of hair styling salons. Aaron Sr. ran the business, while his wife and children were all stylists. At 26, Aaron moved to Los Angeles where he worked as a hairdresser and began to design wedding gowns and other special-occasion clothing under his own label, "Michael Aaron." There, Aaron met his lover and best friend Guy Kathcart. They had been living together for 17 years when Aaron died of AIDS.

Making quilt panels in Aaron's memory became a family affair with many long distance phone calls between Guy in Los Angeles and Aaron's parents in Thatcher, Arizona. For one of the panels, Aaron's mother completed the crewelwork on a burlap wicker chair cover that Aaron had set aside years before. With black yarn in a running chain stitch, she sewed his name and the dates he was born and died.

Guy wanted to make a panel of his own for Aaron, using a pair of red silk pajamas Aaron had made for himself. But unable to operate the four sewing machines that Aaron left behind, Guy had to wait for a visit from Aaron's sister, Rebecca Byron, to put the panel together. Rebecca was close to her brother; both she and Guy were at Aaron's side the night he died. During the week they spent working on the panel, Guy and Rebecca shared their memories of the person they mutually adored.

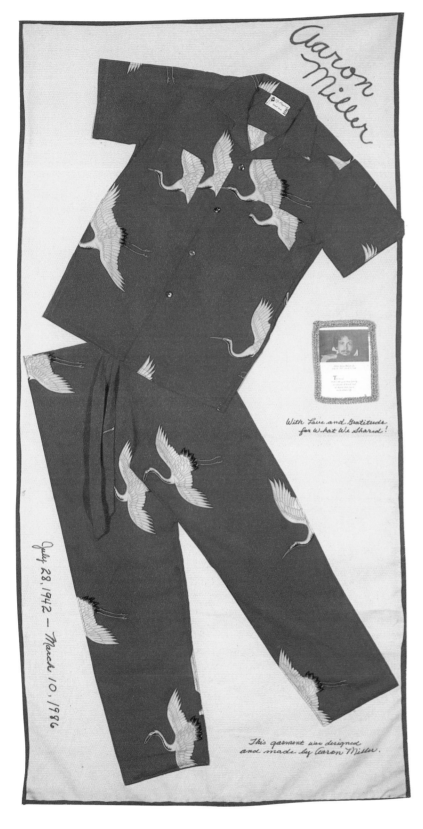

With Love and Gratitude for What We Shared!

July 28, 1942 — March 10, 1986

This garment was designed and made by Aaron Miller.

Aaron John Miller was diabetic and lived most of his life guarding against infections. When the media began informing the public of AIDS, we realized it was a major threat for him.

Our son, Aaron, was gay. This did not separate our Love from him. We Loved our son and he Loved his Mother and Father.

We saw the movie "An Early Frost." A few days later we got the message, Our Son had AIDS! Aaron "Mike" lived another five and a half months before he died. He took one day at a time, taking each day with gratitude for having lived 43 years.

He left a loving family, a loving companion and many friends . . . We Love You, Mike!

Mother and Dad

Aaron's lover and sister sewed this panel together. In small print under the photograph of Aaron, they included the message: "The bond that links your true family is not one of blood but of respect and joy in each other's life."

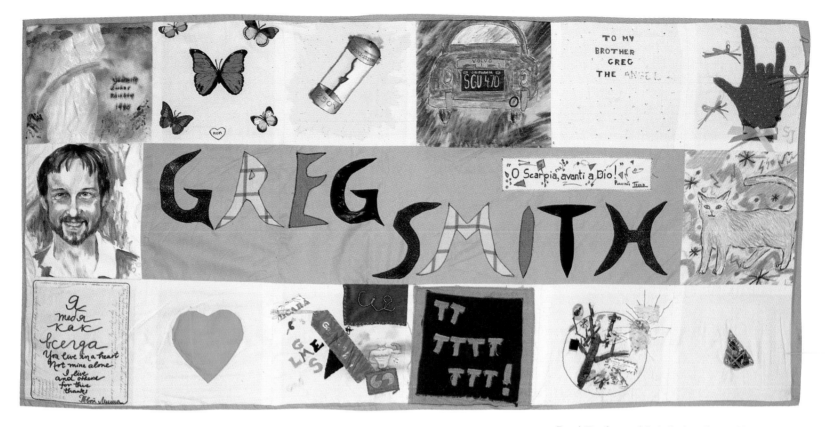

ixteen of the people closest to Greg Smith — his mother, younger sister, ex-lover, friends and coworkers — each worked on a different square of Greg's panel. Then, in Oakland, California, they gathered to sew together their separate squares and remember Greg, an interpreter for the deaf, one more time. It had been almost three years since he died.

Donna, who was at Greg's side constantly through his last year, spelled out his name with the different kinds of fabric he used to wear — denim, flannel, black leather, and, tongue-in-cheek, gold lamé. Donna, who is hearing-impaired, first met Greg at a meeting where he was her interpreter.

A friend who shared Greg's love of opera quoted Puccini's *Tosca*. Duffy, a fellow sign-language interpreter, drew the rear view of Greg's '66 cherry Volvo. Greg's mother glued on delicate butterflies with the word "Mom" written in a heart. His sister embroidered "To my brother Greg, the angel." His friend Dan commissioned an artist to paint a portrait of Greg the way he looked before he became ill. Garet, who interpreted with Greg at the body-building competition for the Gay Games, sewed ribbons and decals from the contests into the panel. With strands of waxed twine, Joe bound a fragment of heavy glass, a souvenir from Greg, to his square. Another friend Lori Beth created an elaborate collage of tree bark, fabric flowers, a kopek, a lock of hair, a cracker-jack he-man, and a paper cutout of Lassie. Sheila, another of Greg's colleagues, quilted a hand in the sign-language gesture for "I love you."

Lori Beth couldn't bring herself to erase Greg's name from her address book. "It's kind of like he's still alive," she says of her friend who died at 34 in December 1984. So instead she cut his name and phone number out of the book and sewed it into the panel. "It was a great way to move it on," she says.

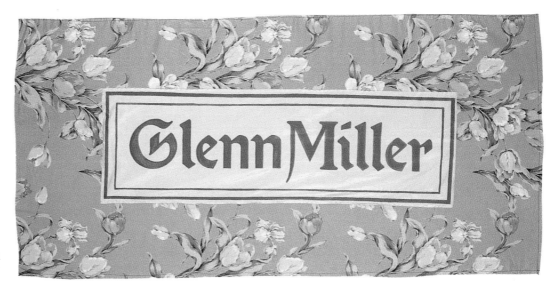

arin Perkins and Glenn Miller were fellow managers at a French bakery in San Francisco. "If provoked," Karin recalls, "Glenn would throw a croissant on the ground and stomp on it." Reminiscing about her friend who died at 31 in 1987, she writes:

He was an obsessive Anglophile and his apartment was filled with Edwardian furniture and coronation ware. One of his greatest pleasures was to put on a tape of Elizabethan music, make tea and scones and have an old-fashioned English tea. He would sit in a chair and pretend he lived in an English cottage and that he had just come in from the village after a little shopping, or in from the garden after staking up the dahlias.

Working in the style that Glenn loved, Karin fashioned his quilt panel out of polished cotton with a traditional British floral pattern. Karin's husband, Shel, lettered the panel in the style of William Morris.

Scenic artist Peter Grote was also inspired by Glenn's love of English Victoriana. The teddy bear represents Glenn's childlike qualities, yellow roses were his favorite flower, and reading and drinking tea were favorite pastimes. "The butterfly came to me in a dream soon after Glenn died," says Peter, "and I knew then that he was all right."

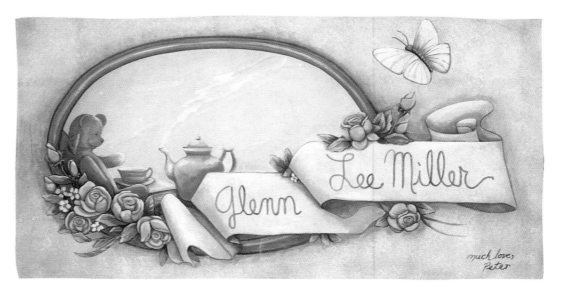

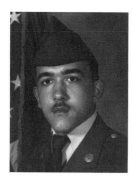

Our Son John A. Politano, Jr., who died of AIDS September 25, 1986, at 3:40 A.M., died at home with MaMa & Daddy at his side, in his room in his Bed with Love & Dignity.

He was an Artist with his oil paint, he was a Poet, he played his Guitar.

His love for Music, Art, Chess, Poetry, Politics & he loved Senior Citizens. (He was Supervisor, Falmouth, Massachusetts.) He donated time to the Elderly.

God bless the Gays & Lesbians.

Love Mr. & Mrs. John & Josephine Politano

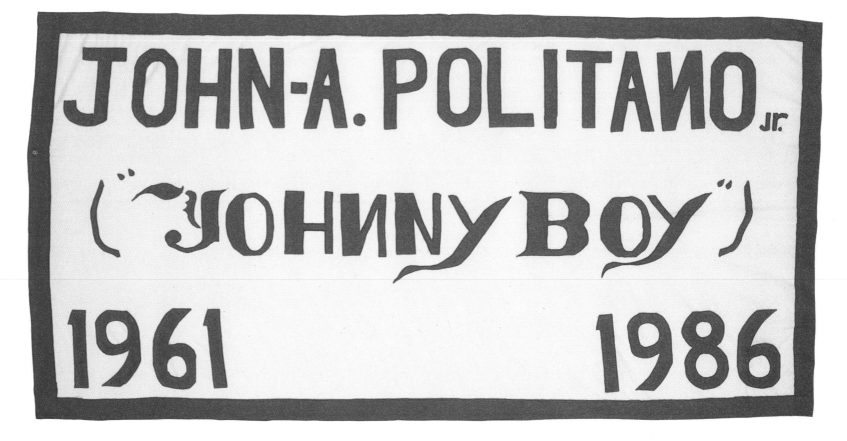

Jim was an inspiration to many people as he fought to live with AIDS. He comforted others and was able to accept the disease as part of God's larger plan. I told him, "You are the strongest, bravest man I know."

I know Love cannot die and Jim's Love surrounds me. He is SOMEWHERE OVER THE RAINBOW with all the many friends who have died with AIDS. They are together and free from pain. Jim, I know I will find you again and we will be together SOMEWHERE.

I LOVE YOU, MY SON.

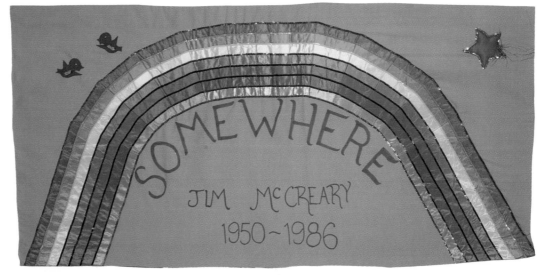

Jim's 15-year-old niece, Tracy, lettered the panel and helped her mother and grandmother with the design. Her 11-year-old sister, Molly, added a wishing star. Recently Tracy comforted a high school friend through the funeral for the friend's uncle, who had also died of AIDS. "We have to worry about it," she says, referring to her fellow teenagers. "We don't want to grow up in a world of fear. It will be our problem a lot longer than it will be everybody else's."

This Thanksgiving, one year since her only son died of AIDS, Mitzi McCreary shared the holiday with a new family. She roasted two big turkeys and opened up her home in Kettering, Ohio, to two other mothers whose sons have AIDS, a mother and father whose son had died recently, and two young men with AIDS whose families had rejected them. "I don't know when I had a nicer day," says Mitzi McCreary, who prepared care packages laden with turkey and pie for her two young guests. "I've lost a mother, a father and a husband, but there is nothing like losing a child. Without the support of the gay community, I could never have made it through this.

"I promised my son that I'd continue working with this disease until they find a cure," says 59-year-old Mitzi, until recently a sales executive for a major hosiery company. "It gets very frightening here in the Midwest. It's scary when you have grandchildren growing up. I know

that my grandchildren are well versed on AIDS, but there are so many others. I want to be the voice for the people who are hurting — for the people who cannot speak out. I guess I'm an activist. I feel like a stronger, more dedicated person for this cause."

When Jim was 19, he attempted suicide and the hospital psychiatrist later told Mitzi the cause: her son was gay. "I was very naive," says Mitzi, who grew up in a small Kentucky town. "I didn't know enough to understand it." Jim battled with his homosexuality, and was so determined to change that at age 21 he underwent 34 shock treatments. His mother, who learned everything she knew about being gay from library books, remembers, "I told him that he had to understand that I loved him, and that his sisters loved him, no matter what. I had to help him accept himself for who he was."

In early 1981, just about the time when Jim really got his life together, he sent his

mother information about a new syndrome then being labeled Gay Related Immune Deficiency (GRID). Jim was working in a hospital in Houston as a respiratory therapist, preparing for a career in anesthesiology. He realized that his bouts of chronic hepatitis could be related to this new disease. Following his subsequent diagnosis, Jim lived with AIDS until November 1986, remaining strong and cheerful for six full years. "Jim was a laugh a minute," recalls his younger sister, Erin. "He kept his wonderful smile and sense of humor through his long illness. He was the most positive force in my life, now and always."

"It feels as if Jim has gone on a trip somewhere," says Mitzi, who chose the songs "Over the Rainbow" and "Somewhere in Time" for Jim's memorial service. "I grieve for each one of the boys that have died, but I know that they're all together, working to fight this disease. I know that they are safe and that they are free."

125

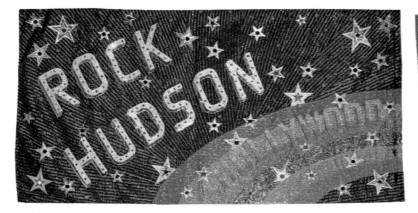

On the back of Rock Hudson's panel, Hollywood designer Warren Caton, who creates custom-made fabric-covered buttons, belts and pleated fabrics for the movie studios, printed, "In remembrance of a true HOLLYWOOD star."

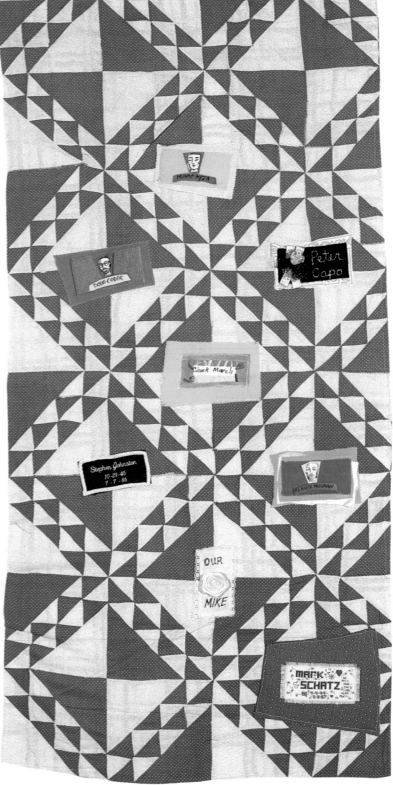

The NAMES Project received over 18 undersized panels, usually three-by-six inches. Volunteers nicknamed these tiny panels, "The Little People."

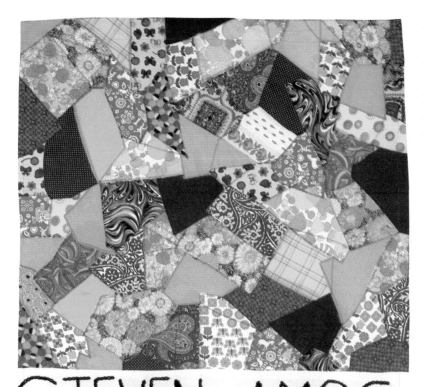

Effie Hemmingsen chose warm colors for the quilt she made to honor her eldest grandson, Steven Amos. A pianist and a visiting nurse, Steven introduced his grandmother to many new adventures, including her first trip to the opera. "We were so close," she says of her grandson who died at 37. "I was there when he was born, and I was there when he passed away."

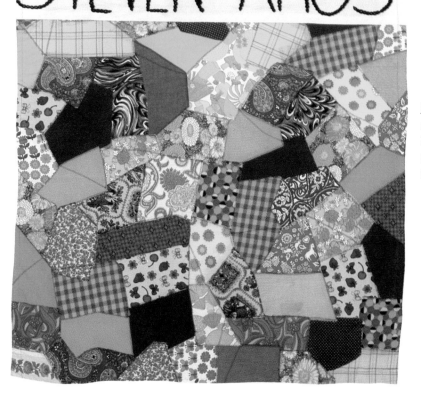

Merle Long's friends, Bob Best and Bryan Pitts, lettered his name on this panel, and then delivered it to the Bodhi Tree Bookstore in Los Angeles, where Merle used to work. The bookstore staff held their own memorial service for the 28-year-old salesclerk, and they each signed the quilt panel in his honor.

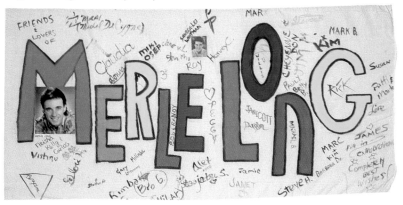

127

After forming a grief support group in San Francisco's East Bay, seven men who lost their lovers and a woman who lost her brother decided to design eight quilt panels for The NAMES Project. Completing their panels separately, they then met at one member's home, removed all the furniture from the living room and laid out their collective work in the exact pattern they wanted. "We put so much of ourselves into them," says Richard Preece of the panels that were later displayed at Mission Dolores Church for the pope's 1987 visit. "We spent three weeks in the group looking at them. It was hard to give them up."

The following stories tell how some of the East Bay quilt panels were made.

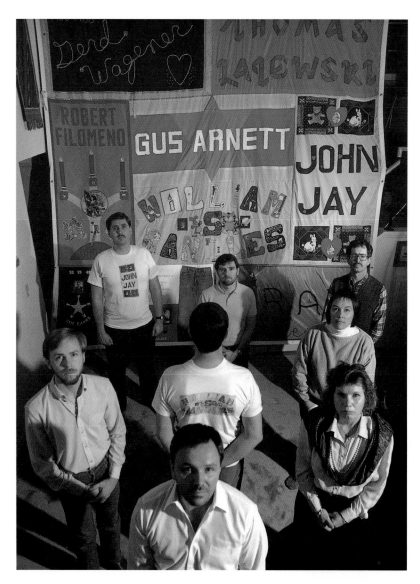

Members of the East Bay grief support group include a professor at a women's college, a high school teacher and a social service administrator. Jerry, the teacher, has turned his back because being gay could cost him his job. "This is the major difference with AIDS and any other death," says Richard Preece, pictured in front. "Jerry had to go through the sickness and death without anyone at work knowing, hiding his grief eight hours a day."

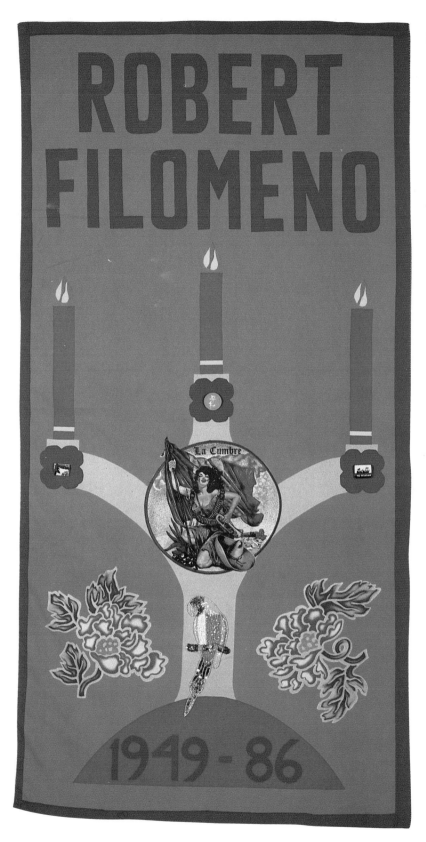

n one of their trips to Mexico, Bob Filomeno and his lover, Jaye Miller, bought an *arbol de la vida* or the Mexican tree of life. Jaye, a professor of history and international studies, found new meaning in this folk-craft piece after Bob died of AIDS in 1986. He stitched the Mexican symbol of rebirth as the central image in the quilt he made in Bob's memory. Then he decorated the tree with buttons from Nicaragua and Hiroshima, and flowers to reflect Bob's love of nature. The yellow ribbon bands on the candles symbolize the revolution in the Philippines and the sense of hope it instilled in Bob, who was part Filipino, as he was dying. Jaye also incorporated the motif from Bob's favorite restaurant, La Cumbre. Jaye's ex-wife and her second husband, Rusten, helped him with the quilt as did Deborah Martin, one of Bob's best friends. The members of the East Bay Support Group provided the bolstering Jaye needed to complete the task. "I've grown to trust these people more than anything," he says.

Bob, a former administrative assistant at U.C. Berkeley's Student Health Services, was surrounded by his family when he died: his mother, his sister and his four brothers. "He radiated love and respect," writes Jaye. "Because both our families loved us very much, they came to understand that our relationship was very similar to that of a married heterosexual couple. Being homosexual, you don't get that same recognition in society. There's that in-between place where you don't know where you stand and how much you can say. Even I partly denied how important our relationship really was. In the last year, we became much closer to each other. There was a revelation and a tremendous growth — a tremendous depth of awareness. He came to know how much I really loved him, and I didn't know, until he became ill, just how important our relationship was to me."

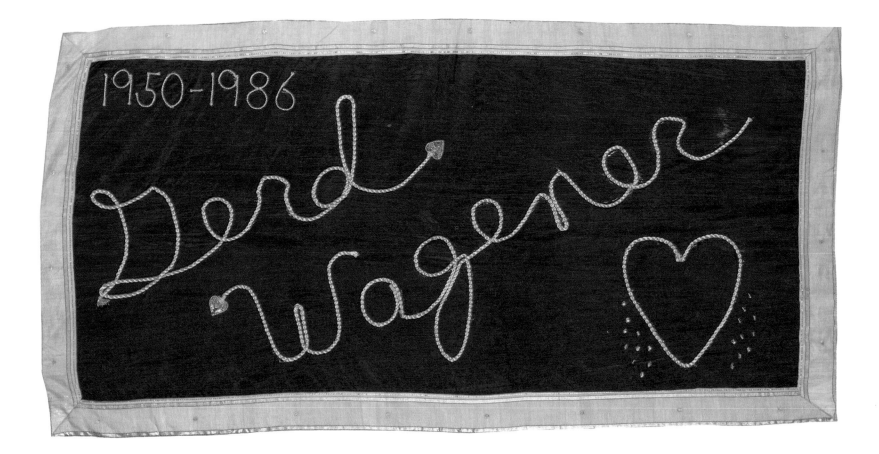

 don't know why I'm alive and he's dead," says Richard Preece of his lover, Gerd Wagener. "I've watched so many people who were healthy die, and I'm still here."

Gerd and Richard met in Europe, and lived there for a year before moving to the Bay Area. Gerd, who is from Belgium, was completing his law degree. They first began talking about AIDS in 1982 when Richard was diagnosed with lymphadeno-pathy, a possible precursor to AIDS. In July 1985, they took Richard's 62-year-old mother, who had never been to Europe, on a trip to Paris. Gerd, who had been suffering from night sweats, constant infections and abnormal fatigue for almost a year, stopped in at the Pasteur Institute, one of the leading clinical centers for AIDS. Four months later, Richard was hospitalized for congenital heart failure. Although he had not been given a positive AIDS diagnosis, his lungs were filled with fluid, and he was placed in the AIDS ward. When he came home, he suggested a double suicide. Gerd, who was determined to have a normal life, tried to assure Richard that it was all a bad dream, and that they would grow "to be little old men together."

The next three months were very special. "All the petty day-to-day stuff falls away, and only the love remains," says 41-year-old Richard. "What's left is a tremendous awareness of your feelings for each other and an appreciation for what you have."

Just before Christmas 1985, Gerd, a gourmet cook, spent three days preparing a grand holiday dinner for their friends. The day after, he collapsed. Hospitalized twice in January, he still mustered the strength to drive Richard, who was struggling for breath, to the hospital on February 14. A suffocating rash had spread down Richard's throat. Gerd was too weak to visit Richard, and when he tried to fetch him from the hospital several days later, he collapsed in the driver's seat of their car. "We found ourselves at home, neither of us able to take care of ourselves or each other," remembers Richard, who was out of his mind with fever, fear and pain. Richard's mother arrived from San Diego to help, and friends came by to clean the house, wash the windows, walk the dogs, and make trips to the pharmacy. Four days after Richard returned from the hospital, he had to take Gerd back to intensive care, where Gerd, then 35, died 48 hours later.

"I went into hibernation for a year," Richard says softly. "Gerd was the first person in my life that I really knew loved me, and it was devastating to watch him die. I couldn't be around people. I didn't know what to say. I couldn't talk — until I joined this loving, caring support group. I

don't like the idea of focusing my life around grieving, but the people in this group have become close friends. They understand why I can't just pick up the pieces and go on.

"I do fine alone, but it is not my choice. I don't dare do anything long-term. All of us in the group are used to being couples, sharing decision making, and sleeping with someone. We all want it again. The other side, however, is terrified of reinvolvement, abandonment and loss again. Although I have wonderful support from my family, I'm lonely — not for friends, but for the intimacy that we had developed in a ten-year relationship. I don't have ten years anymore. Besides, who wants to be involved with someone who is HIV positive and has health problems?

"When Gerd died I lost my lover, my best friend, mentor and business partner," says Richard, who continues to run their property management business and carry out their mutual plans for renovations of their home in Berkeley. Gerd's paintings and photographs still hang on the walls. "I don't want anyone disturbing 'our home,'" says Richard. The only room he could no longer live with was the den, where they used to sit every evening in the two leather chairs, reading or listening to music. "I couldn't bear to sit with that empty chair next to me," he says. "But the house is a bit of a shrine. I have made those aspects of him that I value a part of me. Even though he is dead, everything he was continues to influence my perceptions and behavior. I see and experience everything now through his eyes as well as my own.

"I have a level of seriousness that I never had before. I've made a lot of changes in my life. I don't spend energy on people or activities I dislike. I don't float through anything — I really treasure being alive. I have this tremendous urge to take life and live it because we may not have much time left. I've seen too much death, and seen too many people die so suddenly.

"I wanted Gerd's panel to be simple and

elegant," he adds. "Gerd was a reserved, private man, and I wanted the panel to be something he would approve of. He was an intellectual, an avid reader and an historian. He spoke six languages, loved to cook, enjoyed classical music and opera, and brought refined taste to our home. Creating this panel was a very big process for such a simple thing because it is a reflection of him and of me."

In gold rope, Richard signed his lover's name, Gerd Wagener, on the forest-green taffeta panel. The 10 gold teardrops on either side of the gold rope heart represent the 10 years Gerd and Richard spent together. Richard fabricated a border of Indian silk from a sari belonging to the mother of a close friend.

"I thought that if I made it through one year, it would all be better," he says. "But grief doesn't just evaporate. Even now, after almost two years without him, it is hard to want to go on. My security in the love we shared sustains me. I treasure our ten years together and will keep him alive in my heart and mind forever."

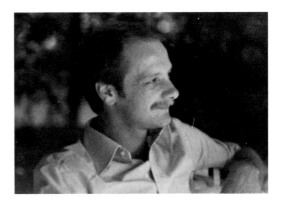

After Gerd Wagener (above) died, his lover Richard took his ashes to his family in Belgium. Gerd's mother took Richard in as the son she had lost.

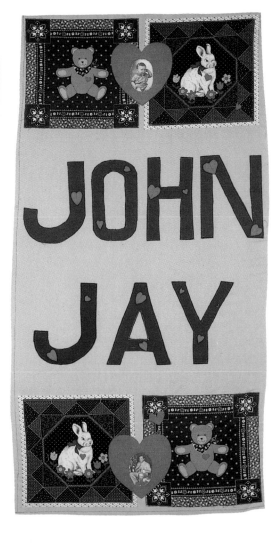

red Canning wanted to create a memorial for his lover of five years, Gus Arnett, without any assistance. But the panel only came together at a potluck dinner at The NAMES Project when friends got involved. Fred took his 12-year-old son shopping for fabric, and the mother of a close friend did the final sewing.

Bright and startling, the quilt honoring Gus, a former engineer, represents his vitality and energy. Fred's son had a special relationship with Gus — they'd go shopping together on Saturday mornings, change the oil in the truck, and go to the dump. Gus, who died at 41 in 1986, was ill for 15 months, and Fred would bring his children to the hospital to visit. After Gus died, Fred's two teenage daughters and his son spent every weekend with their father to comfort him through some difficult months.

ob glued two photographs to his lover's panel — a photo of John Jay as an infant and a photo of him before he died. Bob made the panel at The NAMES Project workshop, then took it home and laid it on John's bed. This was the first time Bob had a sensation of John's presence since his death. Later, Bob and his East Bay Support Group comember Jerry held a ceremony at their church where they blessed the banners they had made for Bill Randles and John Jay.

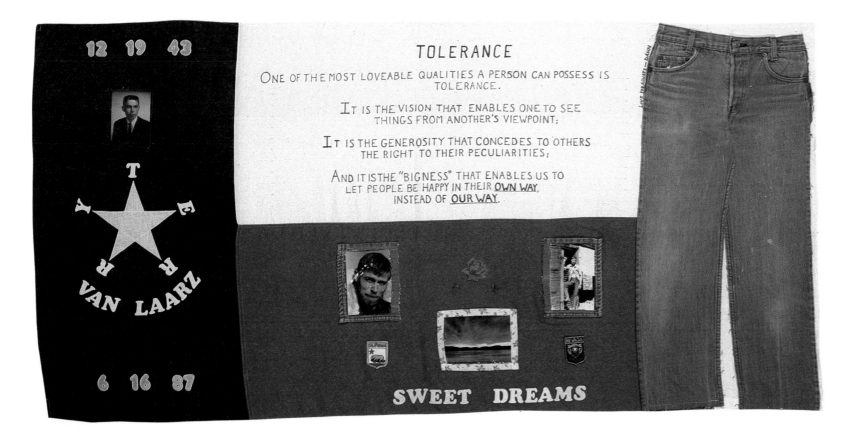

TOLERANCE

ONE OF THE MOST LOVEABLE QUALITIES A PERSON CAN POSSESS IS TOLERANCE.

IT IS THE VISION THAT ENABLES ONE TO SEE THINGS FROM ANOTHER'S VIEWPOINT;

IT IS THE GENEROSITY THAT CONCEDES TO OTHERS THE RIGHT TO THEIR PECULIARITIES;

AND IT IS THE "BIGNESS" THAT ENABLES US TO LET PEOPLE BE HAPPY IN THEIR OWN WAY, INSTEAD OF OUR WAY.

SWEET DREAMS

arly in his adult life, Terry devised his own "creed of tolerance," a philosophy that was articulated in a poem that he carried around in his wallet. Whenever Terry made new friends, he would take the poem out and show it to them.

Terry showed the poem to Dáhn van Laarz soon after they met at a bar in Reno. Terry, then 41, had already been diagnosed with AIDS and told Dáhn that he wanted to live out all his dreams before he died. As their friendship grew Dáhn, who was 16 years younger than Terry, taught Terry how to fish and how to ride a motorcycle. With matching Suzuki bikes, they took frequent camping trips to fish for trout in the mountain streams above

Reno. Terry's last name had been King while growing up in a farming town outside Amarillo, Texas. But he and Dáhn held a marriage celebration in May 1985 and Terry legally changed his name to match his lover's.

The fishing flies that Dáhn incorporated into Terry's panel are from the couple's last camping trip. "He wanted me to show him all my favorite things," says Dáhn, who now lives alone with Zuki, the cat he and Terry named after their motorcycles. "It was important for him to allow me to have memories of him."

Dáhn carried Terry's ashes on the back of his motorcycle and, with Patsy Cline's "Sweet Dreams" playing in the background, he scattered them at Lake Tahoe.

Dear Terry,

I've tried to show some of the facets of you in this panel, some of the things that were close to your heart. There's a pair of your favorite Levi's, a rose, fishing flies, and various photographs: high school graduation so very long ago, your portrait that sunny winter's day we were out on the motorcycles, last fall at that old mining shack that reminded you of rodeo days, and Lake Tahoe at sunset, may you rest there in peace.

Loving you always, Dáhn and Zuki-cat.

P.S. All those empty areas? Maybe I couldn't fill them in and complete things for the same reason your earthly life couldn't be complete — lack of time. Whatever isn't there, just be aware that my love is.

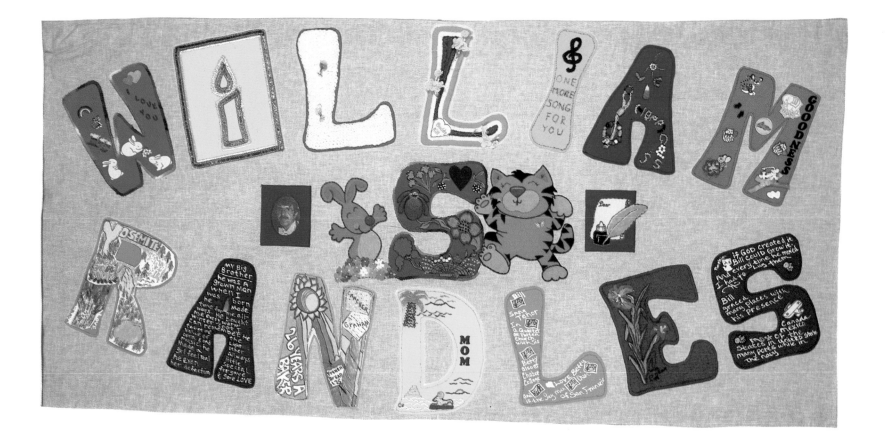

134

ach letter of William Randles's name was designed by a different person in his life, including Jerry, his lover of 19 years, Jerry's children from a prior marriage, their neighbors, choir group and congregation members, Bill's mother and his sisters. Jerry decorated the letter "W" with a rainbow-colored 19 to represent their 19 "colorful years of ups and downs."

Vivian and Teresa from Jerry and Bill's church wrote a note to Jerry saying, "Our tears of memory color Bill's 'I' and he will be in our hearts forever. Love you both." A neighbor, Inez, knitted the "L," and added two wineglasses for the many times that she and Bill sat in his yard, sharing drinks and gossip. The second "L" was decorated with dandelions by Vickie, another neighbor who first met Bill when he came into her garden to pick dandelions from her lawn. The heart that says "Buddy Bill" is from Jason, Vickie's three-year-old son.

Kim, who sang with Bill in the Chabot College choir, outlined the "I" with thread taken from the fringe of a scarf Bill had given her one wintry day.

For many years Jerry's children accompanied their father and Bill on holidays. When they reached high school, Allison and Mark moved in with Bill and Jerry. Allison drew a spider on top of the "A," recalling how Bill would try to save them when she wanted to kill them. She added macramé because Bill had taught her how to do it. The letters below the spider represent the times that Bill helped her with her spelling and her schoolwork. Mark and his wife Pamela made the "M." Bill was best man at their wedding and the wedding favor is from this. The pink and blue baby elephant is a token from Bryan, the infant grandson that Bill hoped for but never met.

Bill and Jerry's friend Leslie, an artist, incorporates a rabbit and tiger motif in

everything she makes for them. Leslie painted these Chinese animal symbols corresponding to their birth years on the "S."

Bill's sister Carla decorated the "R," the "A" and the "N." On the pine tree next to the campfire in the letter "R," Carla painted Bill and Jerry's initials. She decorated the "N" to recall the 26 years Bill baked cookies and crackers for Sunshine Bakery. Bill's mother painted a palm tree and sunset on the "D" to recall a holiday in Hawaii. Bill and Jerry took both their mothers as well as Mark, Allison and a nephew on this trip. Betty, a sister, dedicated the letter "L" to Bill's music. On the "S" she wrote, "If God created it, Bill could grow it. And every time he moved I had to lug them." Bill's niece Carol embroidered flowers on the "E" for the many hours Bill spent with his plants.

In the center of the panel, Jerry added a scroll with a quill and ink for all the letters Bill wrote to gay prisoners. The photograph of Bill was taken on Mark and Pamela's wedding day.

After 16 years together, Bill and Jerry arranged a Holy Union service to announce their love for each other to God and to the world. Bill wanted his family to stand with them at the communion but they refused and he never saw them again. He longed to reconnect with his family, and wrote many letters that never got mailed. The day he was diagnosed with AIDS, Bill asked Jerry to contact his family. His mother arrived at his hospital bedside the next day and remained with him until he died three days later. His sister Carla admits that she couldn't bring herself to go to the hospital to visit her brother because she was afraid of catching AIDS. Over the telephone, Bill forgave her and gave her his love. She ends her inscription on the letter "A" with an apology for not being with him those last few

days. Bill's brother and sisters were getting dressed to visit him the morning that he died.

At Bill's memorial service, the family made up for the ceremony they missed. This time they stood with Jerry as he took communion. Now they have drawn even closer to Jerry. They worked on the quilt with him and he always stops off in Stockton to see them whenever he visits Bill's grave. Often he arrives with his son, daughter-in-law and grandson in tow. Bill loved kids, and Bill and Jerry dreamed of growing old together, retiring and enjoying their grandchildren.

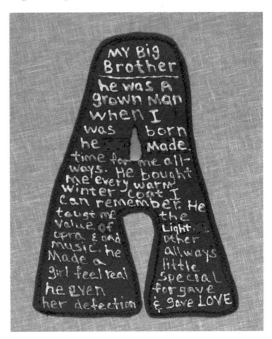

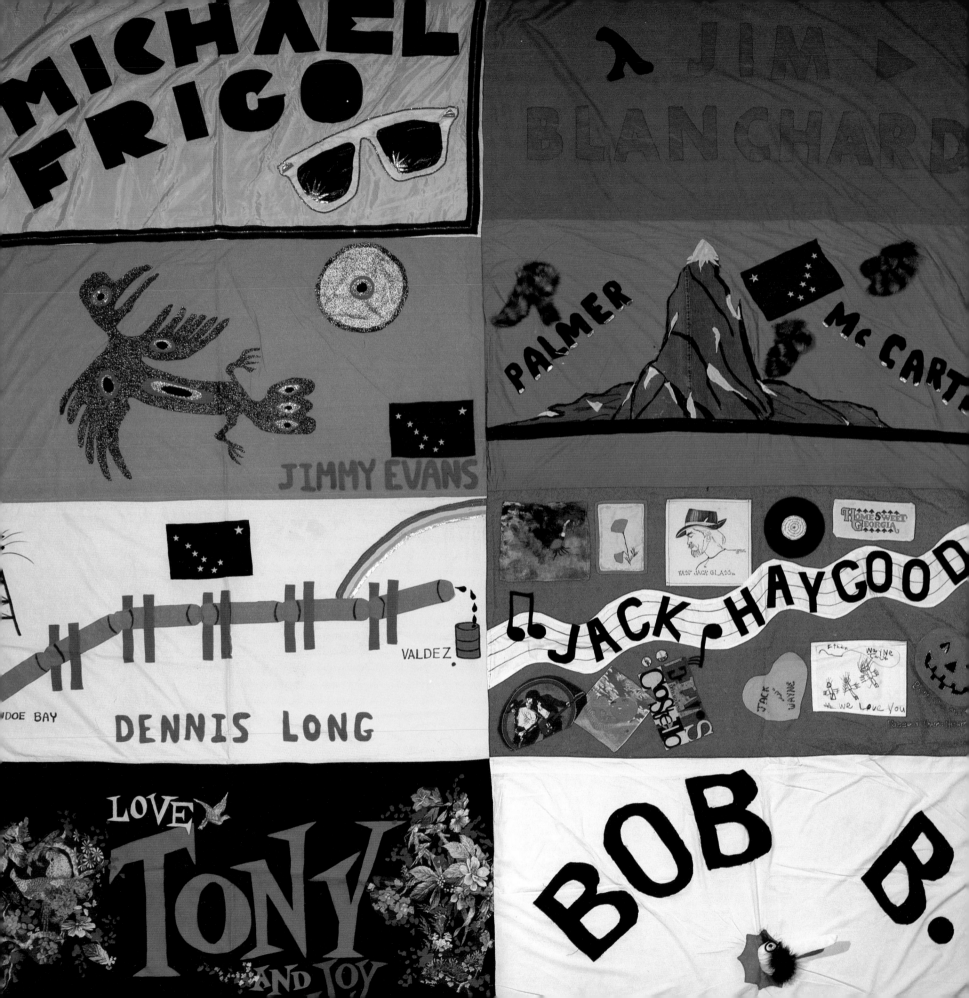

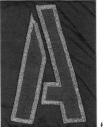

t 1:00 A.M. on October 11, Rod Shelnutt wakes up in a noisy dorm room at Georgetown University, straps on his fanny pack, stuffed with wire cutters, plastic cable ties and his camera. Mark Kroll gets ready as if he were going on a date. He showers, splashes on cologne, and irons his clothes. Seth Miller and Steve Sim hail a cab to the Washington Mall.

At 1:30 Ron Cordova and Mike Bento, the site logistics coordinator, run through the final checklist: portable generator, gas, 125 boxes of programs, volunteer caps and badges, television monitors, electrical cable, brooms, rope, food and The Quilt.

It's 1:45 when The NAMES Project fleet, including a 24-foot truck, a 33-foot Winnebago, and a pickup truck with a four-ton scissor lift in tow, pulls out of the Georgetown University parking lot. The caravan winds through Washington, past the Watergate and onto the Capitol Mall.

By 2:00 A.M. the volunteers on the mall in the dark with flashlights, walkie-talkies, clippers, grommets, ties and rolls of walkway fabric, begin to create the grid. The night is clear. The grass is thick and there is a heavy dew. Two volunteers roll out sheets of plastic to protect The Quilt. Flashlights flicker all over the mall as they work through the early hours of the morning.

Around 5:00 people start to panic. They aren't even halfway through laying the grid down yet, and there are only two hours left until sunrise.

At 6:45 the gridwork is complete. Everyone is stunned at its sheer magnitude and beauty. But to Ron, it looks exactly the way he had envisioned it when he started designing months ago. He had paced it out so many times. It is the same length as the distance from Café Flore to the front door of The NAMES Project. He smiles as he thinks back to all the nights he lay awake worrying that he may have missed one panel, which would throw the whole grommeting system into disarray. The volunteers hurry to place folded quilts in the center of each grassy square just in time for the opening ceremony.

At 7:00 A.M. the set up team hold hands tightly in a circle. "We did it!" Cleve says softly.

It's 7:10 and four teams of eight are at opposite ends of The Quilt, standing in circles around the first four squares to be unfolded. They clasp hands and look at one another, shivering in the brisk morning chill. Rod Shelnutt, the captain of unfolding team D, looks east at the huge red sun rising above the Capitol. "It's the most perfect sunrise I've ever seen," he says to himself.

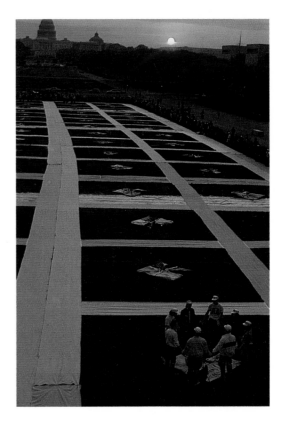

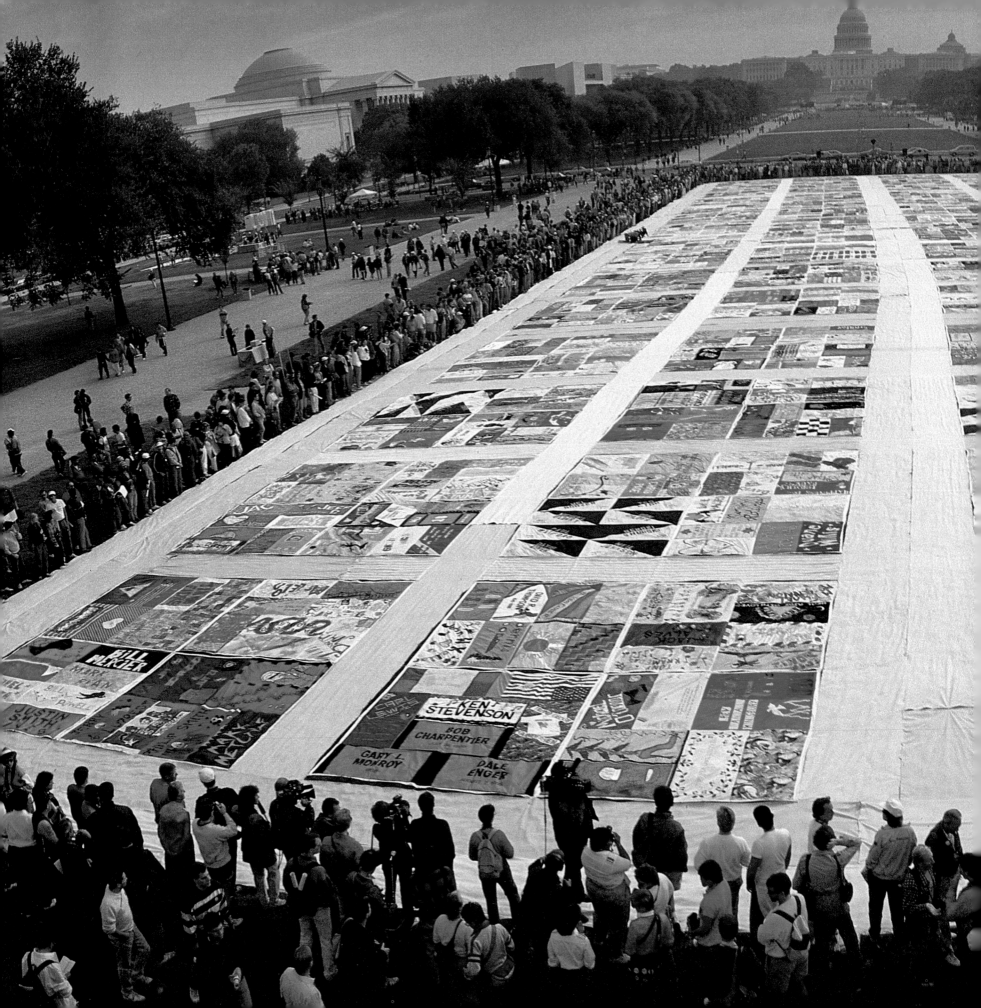

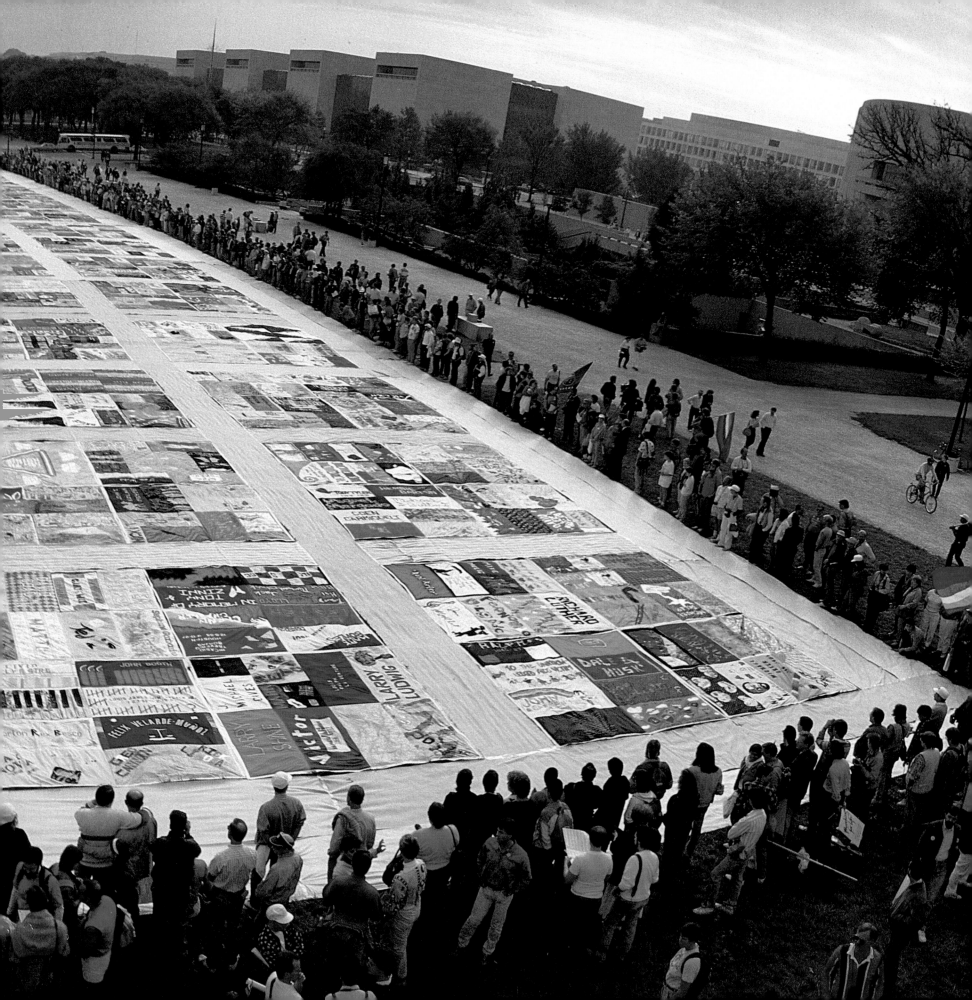

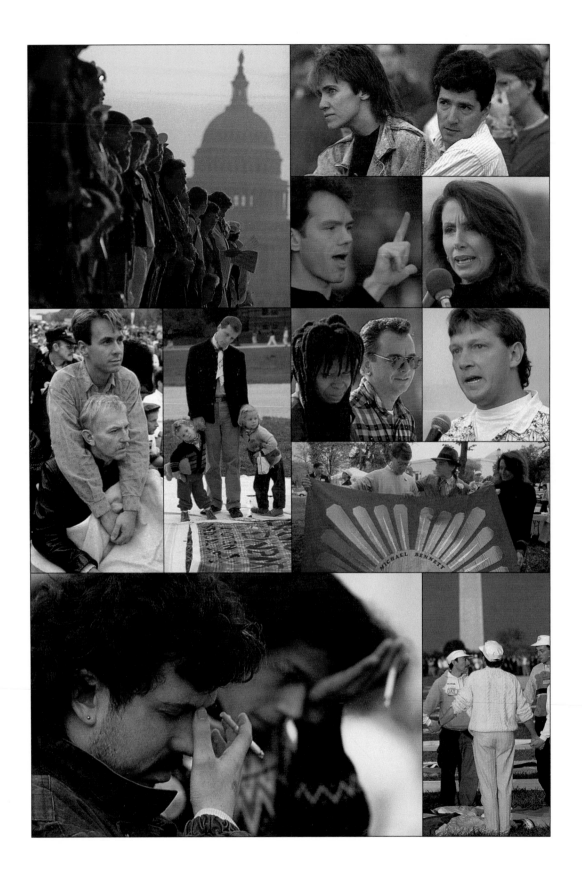
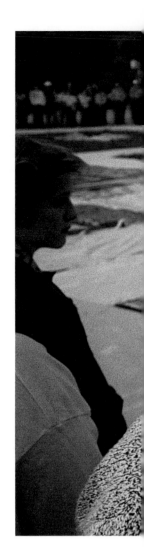

140

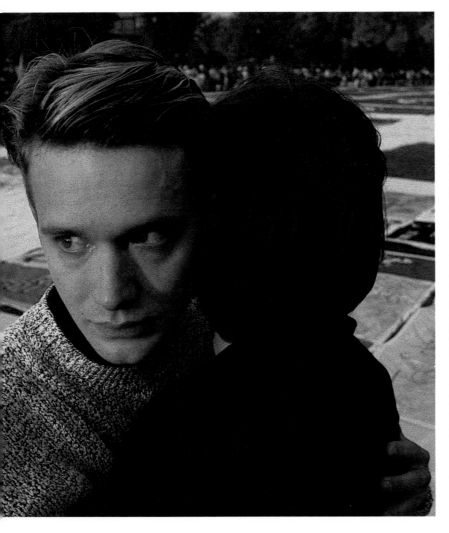

At 7:13, just as the early shafts of daylight stream down on the Capitol Mall, stage manager Paul Hill escorts Cleve Jones to the podium. Facing the U.S. Capitol building, with the white fabric skeletal gridwork of The Quilt laid out on the grass behind him, Cleve starts reading the first 32 names of people memorialized in The Quilt. "Marvin Feldman," he reads forcefully into the mass of microphones. Marvin, his dearest closest friend. Here it was, only a year since Marvin died, and they had talked about the remote possibility of this project together not long before that. Now, standing between the Capitol building and the Washington Monument, Cleve reads the names slowly and deliberately, pausing purposely between each. His voice breaks as he reaches the end of his list, and as he steps off the podium, he collapses into a friend's arms and weeps.

A crowd of 1,500 gathers silently on the outside edge of the white fabric gridwork, as 60 celebrities, politicians, parents and AIDS activists take turns reading the roll call of names. Among the readers are actor Robert Blake, Merv Silverman, the executive director of AMFAR (American Fund for AIDS Research), actor-playwright Harvey Fierstein and U.S. Representative Nancy Pelosi, who ends her list with "my sweet Suzy" for her niece Susan Piracci Roggio who is remembered in The Quilt.

The four unfolding teams open sections of The Quilt one by one as the names are being read. The 24-foot square blocks open like petals of a flower, revealing the colors of 32 individual panels. Lifting the open quilt, then rotating it into place — turning like a pinwheel — the unfolding team kneels down to attach the squares to the walkways with the plastic ties stuffed in their pockets. The materials of some of the panels are so light that when the unfolders lift The Quilt, it just floats. The four teams alternate from opposite ends of The Quilt, zigzagging toward each other.

The names go on and on and on. Jack Caster's powerful voice can be heard all the way to the Washington Monument. "I made sure that every name would be heard," says Jack. When Sue Caves, president of Families Who Care, ends her list with "and my son, J. Michael Caves," a shudder goes through the crowd.

Joseph Papp, producer of the New York Shakespeare Festival, ends with a tribute to "my dear friend and colleague Michael Bennett." Then, in front of photographers, with his wife Gail at his side, Papp unties the satin ribbons of the red fabric roll under his arm and holds up a shimmering quilt panel emblazoned with Michael Bennett's name and a metallic sunburst, the design from the finale of Bennett's stellar production, the longest-running Broadway musical, *A Chorus Line*. The N.Y. Shakespeare Company's properties department spent two days putting the quilt panel together. Papp walks over to the panel check-in area and turns it in with all the other panels that continue to arrive through the day.

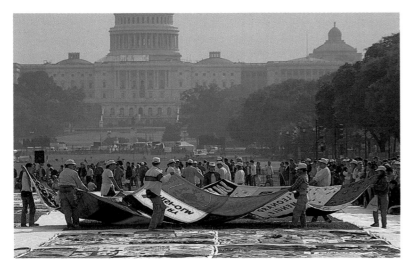

While standing on the podium reading names, Deane Dixon holds the panel for her 31-year-old son Rick who had died only a month earlier. For just a moment she worries that her panel is too simple after seeing all the others.

It takes over three hours for the 60 squares to be laid out, as each empty block of green is filled with the vivid colors of the quilt. As Mike Smith reads the last set of names, the 50-foot-long signature sash is rolled down the middle of The Quilt, which covers two city blocks. The crowd is hushed. Out of the silence, one man sobs uncontrollably. Cleve, Mike and Ron join the unfolders as they hug, cry and sign The NAMES Project signature sash.

Whoopi Goldberg pushes Jim Maness, a longtime friend with AIDS, in a wheelchair around The Quilt. Young parents with strollers, clutching their children, wander up and down the network of walkways. A little boy in a yellow slicker gets on his hands and knees to pat the panel made out of quilted pinwheels. A man arrives with his lover's ashes in a plastic bag and places them on his panel. Entire families search for names. Many bring bouquets of flowers and mementos to lay on the quilt panels. A mother points out a panel to her toddler son. "See, his name is Michael, too," she says to him. "He died of AIDS, remember, we talked about that?" Two deaf men are signing to each other. Both are crying. "Walking through the panels is so much like being in a cemetery," says Woody Moseley, a 40-year-old psychiatrist. "But it's very different. It also feels alive. I am as moved by the people who came to see the quilt as I am by my own feelings and the panels." People are crying unabashedly, comforting one another and strangers.

A middle-age couple approaches Christopher Hausen, a 54-year-old NAMES Project volunteer. "This is the first homosexual event we have ever been at," the man says to Christopher. "Our son has a panel here. Now we understand homosexual people in a new way."

"The Quilt is a mass of humanity and everybody who came to the Washington display was just so loving," says Richard Wagner. "If everyone could have been here today, it's hard to believe there could be any hatred left in the world."

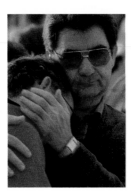

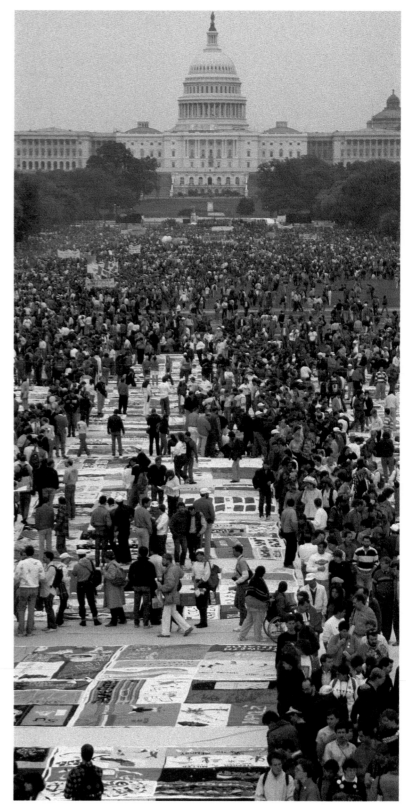

142

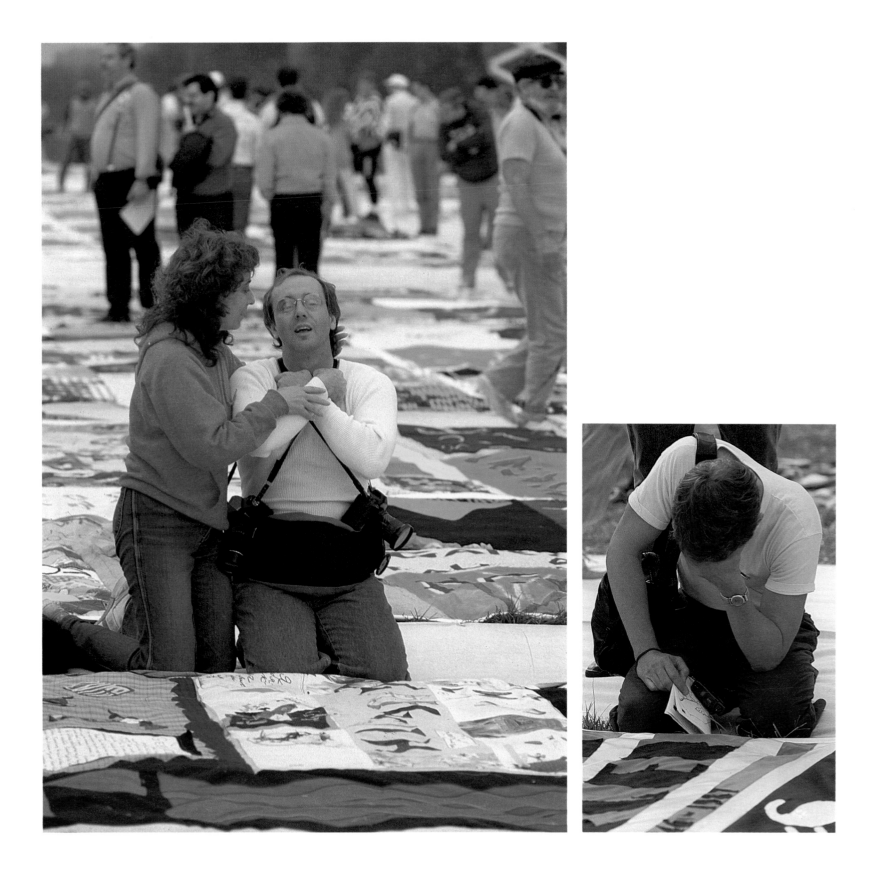

Seven members of the East Bay Support Group arrived at the Washington Mall at sunrise for The Quilt's unveiling ceremony. They found the spot where their panels were to be unfolded. Jerry and Bob, wearing T-shirts with color xeroxes of their panels for Bill Randles and John Jay respectively, embraced the other members of their group and wept as their quilt was opened and their lovers' names read. They cried in each others arms for 15 minutes as names echoed around them.

Ann Des Rosiers and her husband Jerry drove to Washington from Worcester, Massachusetts, with Thom and Kenny, two home-care workers who helped Ann look after her son Anthony Ferraro. Thom, Kenny and Anthony's nurse Sue pinned a note and a "caring ribbon" on his quilt panel. "The ceremony was done with such dignity," says Ann who made many new friends on The Quilt. "I felt that my son wasn't alone."

Brian O'Sullivan traveled to Washington from Chicago to see the panel he made for "Little Ronnie" Reynolds. He had to return home almost immediately because he was feeling so ill. He died one month later.

Arla Ellsworth, whose husband of 22 years died of AIDS, went with 15 members of her bereavement group to see The Quilt. She didn't feel comfortable joining in the Lesbian and Gay Rights March, but she watched from the sidelines. "I stood with all these gay men," she recalls, "and I knew that I hurt just as bad."

Keith Gann, who has AIDS, walked around the periphery of The Quilt alone. "How much more can we take?" he wondered. The panel he had made for junior high school teacher Paul Rohrer from Council Bluffs, Iowa, was with the others now.

Jim Swope saw the completed quilt for his lover Chuck Morris for the first time when it was laid out on the Capitol Mall. When he found the panel, he wanted to touch it, but it was out of reach. Just as he was feeling most alone, his sister arrived. Later in the day, Jim returned to Chuck's panel. Again he wasn't prepared for the power of The Quilt. This time, he took off his shoes, crawled out to the panel to touch it and to say good-bye one more time.

Jerry Mangan took the train from Provincetown with his girl-friend and daughter to see The Quilt, to hear his brother Nick's name read, and to be part of the march. It was a difficult day for Jerry because the event was so public and what he had been through with Nick was so intensely private. That morning, Jerry looked at himself in the mirror, wondering if he would have his brother's courage facing his own death. "I'm thankful to him for his love, his courage and his forgiveness," says Jerry. "May his spirit be reborn in a land where men and women are not persecuted for their individual natures."

And after everyone had gone home, late at night with the Capitol and the Washington Monument lit up on either end, the impression of The Quilt's grid was still left on the lawn.

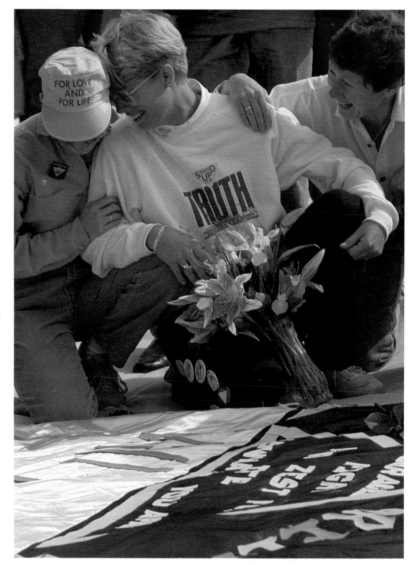

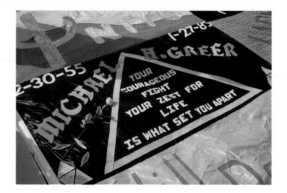

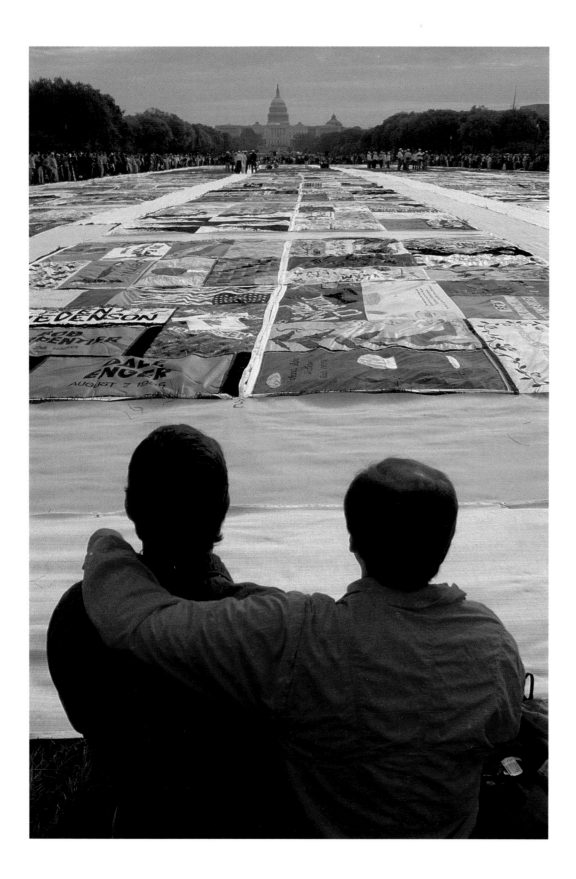

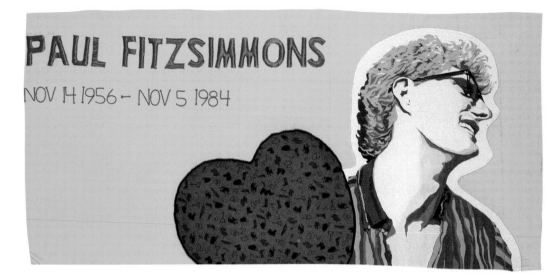

NOV 14 1956 – NOV 5 1984

Paul Fitzsimmons, a secretary for a legal firm in New York, spent winters skiing with his lover David Aurand and their close friends Kathleen Cheetham and Dorene Davis. Kathleen, Dorene and Jill Cooper, Paul's sister-in-law, designed these matching panels for David and Paul who died one year and five months apart. Dorene attempted to capture Paul's free-spirited nature in this portrait. She copied a photograph of Paul, snapped by David, sitting in the back seat of a convertible with his hair blowing in the wind.

The following names represent the panels displayed in Washington, D.C. in October 1987. Panels that appear in this book are indicated by the corresponding page number. An asterisk indicates that the panel was not part of The Quilt when it was displayed in Washington.

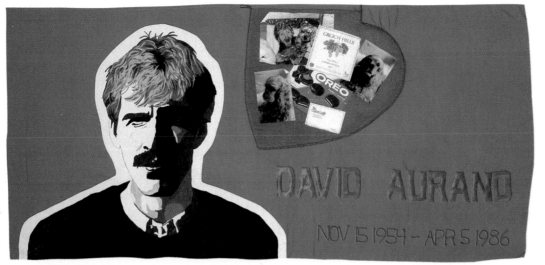

Kathleen took the photograph of David used for this portrait on the ski slopes of Heavenly Valley. It was taken the day they scattered Paul Fitzsimmons's ashes. Dorene included his business card in this memorial because David, a wine steward at the Quilted Giraffe restaurant in New York, loved his job. When David became ill, the Quilted Giraffe owners moved him into an apartment above the restaurant where they were able to care for him.

Bob Borelli
Nicasio Trevenio Borjas
Michael Borno
Dan Borntrager
Brent Borrowman
Justin Bostwick
Dan Bowers
Michael Bowers
Mark S. Bowles
Roy Bowman
Scooby Bowman
Michael Boyd
Les Boyette
Jim Braden
Bruce Bradley
David Bradley
Francis Brady
Asa Branch
Steve Branson
Douglas Brashears
Richard Brauer
Charlie Braun, *102*
Ralph Bremner
Arthur Bressan
Skip Brewer
Jay Brewster
Michael C. Brians
Tommy Bridges
Raymond Brigham
John Brinson, *67*
Patrick Britain
Richard Brooks
Jay Broussard, *99*
Ben Brown
Bob Brown
Douglas C. Brown
Patrick Claude Brown
Terry Brown
Tom Brown
Tommy Brown
Bill Bucholz
Chuck Buck
Tom Buckingham
Fred Buckley
Brian Buczak
Jerry Bumganner
Gary Buntain
Paul Burdett, *24*
Robert Burger
David Burgess

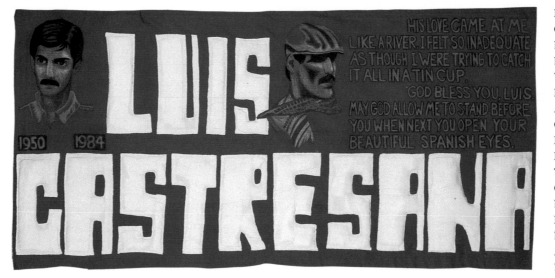

"From the very first, he spoke to me with his eyes," writes Kenneth Rinker of his lover Luis, a professor of languages at the University of Houston. "He looked directly into my eyes, winked and smiled, and with that ushered me into his life."

David R. Burkhart
Bruce Burnett
Bob Bushnell
Roger Buskey
Jim Butcher
Anthony Butler
Michael Buttans
Wayne L. Byers
Charlie Byrd
Bob C.
Jeff C.
John C.
Tom Caddell
Steve Cain
Jim Calderone, *91*
David Calgaro
Peter Callagham
Bob Calvert
Michael Calvert
Ron Camacho
Talmage Camden
Ken Cameron
Bobbi Campbell
David Campbell,* *107*
David C. Campbell
John David Campbell
Robert Lee Campbell, *40*

Wayne Campbell
Daniel Campos
John Canady, *151*
Greg Canning
Peter Capo, *126*
Dan Cappiello
Jon Carberry
Vinnie Cardia
Mark Cardwell
Ron Carey
Ron Carlson
Paul Carlton
Robert Carmal
Coen Carmiggelt
David Caroline
Billy Carson
Steve Carte
Neil Carter
Rocco Cartwright
Luciano Caruana
John Carver
David Cary
Charlie Case
James Martin Case
Raymond Case
Michael Cassidy
Nick Castellano

Joe A. Castillo
Luis Castresana, *148*
Dave Castro
Paul Castro
Tom Castro, *15*
Allen Caswell, *99*
Bill Cathcart
Gregory Catlow
Steve Catron
J. Michael Caves
Ron Cearns
Billy Cerni
Jeff Cerreta
Jorge Cervera
John Chappell
Ronn Charles, *25*
J. Robert Charpenier
Bob Charpentier
John Chatburn,* *113*
Tom Chaudoin
Alan Cherry
Doug Chestnut
Ailekxis Chew
Larry Chisholm
Robert Chodzinski
Queen Christine, *42*
Garry Christofoletti

Gary Christopher
Kyle Citadin
Tony Cius
Rick Claflin
Claude Clark
Gary Clark
Greg Clark
Tom Clark
Richard Clayberg
Scott Cleaver
Stephen Clover
Lowell Clucas
Billy Coates
Lou Cocchiotti
Rick Cochran
Horace Cochrane
Doug Coder,* *126*
Edward Cohee
David Cohen
Ron Cohen
Roy Cohn
Bill Colby
Richard Cole
Gentry Coleman
Joey Coleman
Tod Coleman
Douglas Colesworthy

Michael Collins
Glen Colson
Doug Coner
Danny Conerly
Wm. Connors,* *113*
Mark Connolly
Arthur Conrad, *158*
Charles Cook
Frank Cook
Michael Cook
Tom Cook
Chris Cooper
Danny Corcoran
Fred Corliss
Don Corry
Augie Coton
Lionel Cowan
Howard Cowell
Michael Cowie
Marty Cox
Rick Coyle
Herb Crabtree
Bill Cramer
Jim Crandel
Ken Creel, *39*
Arthur "Rusty" Cregg
Milt Criger
John Crocker
Richard Cromley
Dennis Croteau
Stephen Culp
John Calvin Culver, *37*
Barry Cummings
Charlie Kail
  Cunningham
Robert B. Cunningham
Tom Cunnington
Jonathan Currie
Jonathan D. Currier
Jimmy Curry
Richard Curtis
John T. Cyrus
Emilio D'Antuono
Joe Daerec, *36*
Paul Dague
Gary Dewitt Daloin
Bob Dalterio, *6*
Ed Daly
Dennis Dane
Larry Daniel

Richard Daniel
Guy Daniels
Will Dashiel
Andy Davi
Dennis L. Davis
Mike Davis
Tony Davis
Wade Davis, 36
Jim Dawson
Daryl Day
Kim Day
Alphonse de Laura
David de los Reyes
Francisco de Oyos
Louie de Paolis
Michael de Santis
Doug De Young
Peter Deaett
David Deane
Colin Francis Dearing III
David Deen
Teri Dehn
Fernando Delgado, 67
Kent Delventhal
Chuck Demecs
Ed Denk
Don Denney
George Denney
Pastor Cal Denny
Rick Denton
Joe Depenhart
Bill Depew
Ken Derby
Dennis Dew
Frank Di Gennaro
Paul Diamond, 39
George Dick
Doug Dickinson
Howard Dill
Hal Dillehunt
Rick Dixon, 66
Lyle Dobson
Jane and John Doe, 81
John Doe
Dennis J. Doiron
Gary Dollarhide
Sergio Dominguez
Billy Denver Donald, 98
Buzz Donnelly, 39
Richard Donovan,* 113

Richard J. Donovan
Tom Donovan
Lavelle Dorsey
Stephen G. Dowers
Joe Downing
Lewis Michael Dratt
Charles "Trixie" Drew
Jerry Dreyer
Charlie Drucker
Dan Druid
Frank Drummand
Joe Dubois
Forrest Duke
Nelson Dumlao
Dennis Dunbar
Steven J. Dunn
Dennis Dunwoody
Robert Durkin
George Dutra
Bob E.
Jim E.
Gene Earle
Richard N. Eastman, 99
John Easton
Allan L. Eldridge
Johnny Elizardo
Scott Elliot
John Elliott
Alan Ellis
Morgan Ellis
Robert W. Ellis
Roger Ellis
Steve Ellis
David Emmons
Bruce Engell
Dale Enger
Jaime Enos
Gary Epperly
John Erwin
Roy Esquibel
Marshall Esterson
Allan Estes
Anthony Wayne Estrada
Paul Ettsvold
Jimmy Evans, 136
In Memory of Everyone
Gene Ewins, 33
Tim Eyler
Rod Ezio

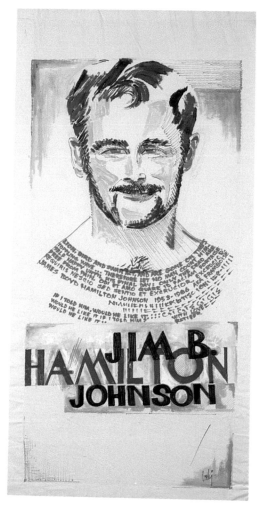

A systems analyst for Pacific Bell, Jim Hamilton Johnson shared a passion for great literature and music with his lover Jay Johnson. Jay adopted Jim who was 19 years his junior, fully expecting Jim to out-live him. "In the panel, his eyes seem slightly crossed," Jay writes. "When he was intent, this did occur."

Gary F.
W. E. F. III
Russell Falcon
Alan Falconer, 15
Wayne Falk
James Famolaro
Tommy Fandal
Emmett Faulkner
Mark Feldman
Marvin Feldman, 19
Randy Feldt
Joe Fernandez, 89
John Fernandez
Larry Fernandez
Anthony Ferraro, 50
Carl Ferreira
John Ferrera
Phillip Ferris
Alan Fiedler
Wayne Field
Mark Fields
Steven Fields
Robert Filomeno, 129
Mark Finch
Michael C. Finden
Herb Finger, 88
Andrew Finochio, 89
Jim Fiore
Tom Fisher
Bob Fiske
Michael Fitzgerald
Paul Fitzsimmons, 146
Rick Flack
Scott Flack
Robert Michael Flaherty
Randy Flanagan,* 20
Jerry Fliegenspan
David B. Fling
Ramon Flores
Michael Flowers
Teddy Fogle
Don Foldon
Tom Foley
Brady B. Fontenot, 99
Mel Foote
Patrick Fortune
Mike Foster
Scott Brian Foster
Michel Foucault, 103
Jean Fournier

Hoy Fowler
Bo Fox
Robert Frakes
Chuck Frank
Jerry Frankel
Norman Frantzen
Joe Fratianni
Mel Freeland
Jay Freezer
Paul Freytag
Richard Bruce Fried, 47
Mike Friedman
Michael Frigo, 136
Rob Frye,* 113
Michael Fuchs
Richard Fuller
Chuck Furbush
Patrick G.
T. G., 99
Terry G.
Tony G.
Bill Gabler
Dr. Claude Gadbois
A. Sydney Gadd III
John Gaffeny, 60
Matsuko Gaffney, 60
Philip Dimitri Galas
Jerry Galbraith
Louie Galicia
Michael Allan Gallanger
Tom Gallegos
Jerry Gallik
Curtis Galloway
Frank Galloway
Dick Gamble
Stephane Garbarino
Steven Garber
Gary Garcia
Richard Garcia
Dan Gardner
Russ Gardner
Dr. John Garner
Jim Garner
Ron Garner
Rick Garrett
Scott Garrison
Xavier Garza
Billy Gassaway
Lou Gaudano
John Gearing

Ray Gearry
Michael Geary
Harvey George
Herman George
Ian Gerard
Michael Gerding
David Germann, *74*
Ron Gertz
Mario Ghelardi
Bradley Gibson
Paul Gibson
John Giebs
Kendrick Gifford
Jack Gilbert
Ralph Ginn
Fred J. Ginsberg
Lyn Joseph Giorgiole
Jack H. Girard
Denis Glas
Jim Gleason
Bill Gluck
Ilja Glusgal
Howard Glyatt
Josh Gniatczynski
David Goad, *39*
Bruce Godfrey
H. Roy Gohl
John Goldring
Steve Gomes
Gary Villa Gomez,* *96*
Amador Gonzalez
Amador Rolando
   Gonzalez
José Gonzalez
Nick Gore
John H. Gosen
Brian Gougeon, *156*
Davie Gracie
Glenn Graeber
Colin Graham
Dennis R. Graham
Timm Graham
Dan Granberg
Tom Grand
Dale Grandstaff
Carl Grant
Tom Graveline
Peter Gray
Joseph Graziano
Tim Green

Bob Greenwood
Ray Greenwood
Robert W. Greenwood, Jr.
Michael Greer
Michael H. Greer
Phil Gregory
John Gretz
Fred Grey,* *20*
Hugh Grey
Milton Griger
Gerald Grunnert
Ron Guilder
Buck Gullett
Trond George
   Gundersen
Larry Gurel
Jose R. Gutierrez
James Guyer
Simon Guzman
Kevin Hain
Mark Halberstadt
Michael Hale
Rob Hale
John Hall
Kip Hall
Ron Hall
Roy Hall
Johnathon Halpern
Jonathan Halpern
John Halpin
James R. Halterman
Jeff Hammock
Pete Hamp
Calvin Hampton
Curtis Hancock
Robert Handel
George Haney
Dale Hansen
George Hansen
John Hanson
Mark Hanson
Walter Hanson
Walter and Mark
   Hanson
Jeff Hardcastle
Grover Paul Hardin
J. Hardin
Shane Harjo
Paul Harkins
Charley Harley

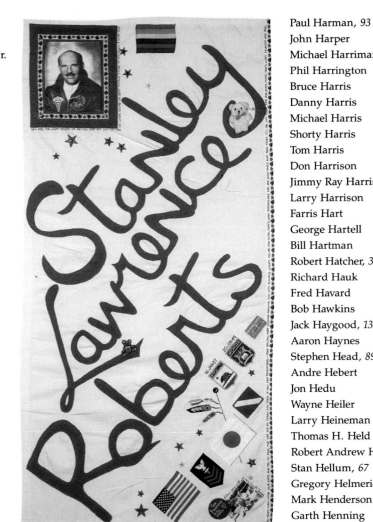

"Stan would say, 'Tommy, you're the best thing that's ever happened to me!' And I'd smile. And I would say, 'Stan, you're the best thing that has ever happened to me!' And we would glow." — Tom Panagiotaros

Paul Harman, *93*
John Harper
Michael Harriman
Phil Harrington
Bruce Harris
Danny Harris
Michael Harris
Shorty Harris
Tom Harris
Don Harrison
Jimmy Ray Harrison, *16*
Larry Harrison
Farris Hart
George Hartell
Bill Hartman
Robert Hatcher, *39*
Richard Hauk
Fred Havard
Bob Hawkins
Jack Haygood, *136*
Aaron Haynes
Stephen Head, *89*
Andre Hebert
Jon Hedu
Wayne Heiler
Larry Heineman
Thomas H. Held
Robert Andrew Heller
Stan Hellum, *67*
Gregory Helmericks
Mark Henderson
Garth Henning
Jon Henrick
Frank J. Henry III
Ahmed Hernandez
Joe Hernandez
Ricardo Hernandez
Bill Herter
Jon Herzstam
Peter Heth, *88*
David Hey
Jesse Hickman
David Hicks
Jim Highland
Jim Hightower
Reggie Hightower, *51*
Arthur B. Hill
Bobby Hilt
Randy Hindman
Duane Hoevet

Duane Martin Hoevet
Abdul Hoffman
Harry Hogerhorst
Jerry Holcomb, *108*
Bryce Holcombe
Rueben Dana Holland
Peter Hollinger
Peter Hollinger, M.D.
Michael Hollister
Michael H. Hollister
Don Holloway
Roland Holstein
Fritz Holt
Joseph Holton
Dennis C. Hook
David Hooper, *38*
Frank Hoover
A. John Horncliff
Roger Hostetler, *6*
James Hotle
Brian Hovey
Donald Howard
Steve Howard
Terry Howell
Tim Howes
Danny Howke
Brian Hoyt
Paul Hubble
Rock Hudson, *126*
Wayne Huff
Chris Hughes
Norman Hughes
Stanley Craig Hugill
Roger Hull
Tom Hunt
Carlos Hunter
Ron Hunter
William Hunter
Charles "Charlie" Hurst
Dale Husk
Dale Hutchins
Stephen Lance Huxtable
Lam Kim Huynh
Allan Hyatt
Richard Ideman
Robert Irizarry
Mort Irwin
Bob Isner
Doug Jabez
Peter Jacklin, *77*

David Jackson
David P. Jackson
David Paul Jackson
Erick Jackson
Paul Jacob
Rick Jacobi
Robin Jacobsen
Tim Jacobsen
Roger Jacoby
Ken James
John Jay, *132*
David Nyle Jenkins
Steve Jenteel
Rodney Jewell
Austin Mark Johnson
David J. Johnson
David Jerry Johnson
Ernest Johnson
Gary Johnson
Jan Johnson
Jerry Johnson
Jim Johnson
Jim B. Johnson, *149*
Kevin Johnson
Kyle Johnson
Michael Magni Johnson
Neil James Johnson
Nina Johnson
Walter Johnson
Warren Johnson
Mark Johnston
Richard Johnston
Stephen Johnston, *126*
Warren Johnston,* *20*
Albert Jones
Bob Jones
Grafton Jones
Ray Jones
Steven W. Jones
Wendell Jones, *44*
Tony Jonson
Milton Davis Jordan
Franz Joseph
Eugene Josephson
Bill Joubert, Jr.
Al Jutzi, *77*
Thom K.
C K III, *83*
Bill Kahler, Jr.
Garth Kalin

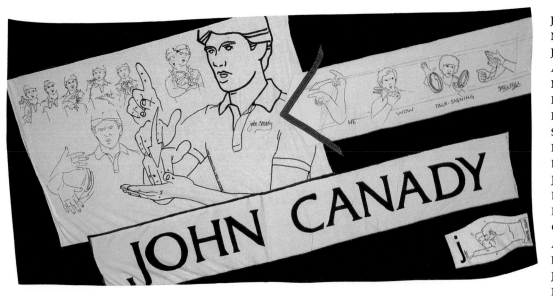

The fifth of eight children in a deaf family, John Canady was the model for two American Sign Language course books. Childhood friend John Smith copied drawings from the books of John signing "okay," "one thousand" and "to walk like a drunk" onto his panel. John Canady was a gifted communicator, able to express himself creatively and dramatically in sign language, a talent comparable to a great singer or storyteller in the hearing world. "Sign-talking…Wow!"

Tim Kane
Joseph Kearns
David Keener
Brian Keith
John W. Kellar
Don Keller
Karl Keller
Scott Kellett
Red Kelly
Sean Kelly
Gregory Kennebeck
Joseph Kenney
Donald Key
Gary Arthur Key, *75*
Tom Keyman
Tony Kiah
Greg Kimberlain
Gary King
Michael King
Mike King
Rev. Randall Kingsbury
Patryk Kinsey
Bob Kissel

Steven Kleckner
Charles "Chaz" Klein
Danny Kludt
Harley Knight
Howard Knopf
Bill Knox, *156*
Alexi Kochs
John T. Kolman
Alex Kovner
Jeffrey Kowalczyk
Warren "Daddy" Kraft
Tony Kramedas
Bill Kraus
David Kreamer
Jeff Kricker
Terry Krueyer
Ken Kuhn
Tom Kulesha
Oggie La Farga
Warren La Follette
Michael LaFrance, *154*
Paul La Marca
Louis Ralph La Venture

Michael Laba
Barron Lafield
Gregory Laird
Jay Lambert, *67*
Michael J. Lamberta
Mark Landsberger
Jay Langan
David Langworthy
Richard Lantz
Richard Lapp
Chuck Larrick
Paul Latchaw
David Lathrop
Dennis Lauriano
Tyrone Lavin
Joe Bob Law
David Lawrence
Thomas Lazewski
Jason James Lazzer
Kurt Le Beau
Victor Le Noble
Roger Dale Leach
Daniel Lee

Jeffrey Scott Leek
Joey Leiset
Don "Parkay" Lemke
Debra Lenard
Reed Lenti,* *28*
Marc Leon
Jessie Leone
Bob Lepley
Dick Lesher
Calu Lester
Ken Lester
Gary R. Leuthauser
Fred Levine
Paul Levinglick
Michael Jay Levy, *21*
Carl Lewis
Michael Lewis
Grant Lighon
Bobby O. Lina
Rick Lindsay
Paul Lindsey
Gary P. Linsky
Geno Linsky

James Lloyd
Neal Lo Monaco,* *60*
Jerry Lo Presti, *77*
Alfred "Al" Lobb
Marco Lodovico
Peter Logan
Ron Lohse
Steve Loignon
Michael Lonergan
Dennis Long, *136*
John Long
Larry Long
Merle Long, *127*
Gary Lonien
Antonio Lopez
Diego Lopez
J. Victor Lopez
Phil Lopez
Victor Lopez
Dennis Lord
Flor Lorenzo
Albert Louie
Clark Lee Lowery
Douglas Lowery
Jeff Lowery
Michael Lowry
Jerry Ludiker
Charles Ludlam
Larry Ludwig
Gustavo Luna
Richard Luther
Jan Patat Luxwolda, *118*
Gary Lybrook
Chuck Lynch
David Lynch
Larry Lynd
Dayna Jo Lynn
Roger Lyon, *34*
Ted Lyon
F. M.
H. L. M.
Tommy M.
W. M.
Bobby Mac Donald
Hank Magdelena
Bart Mahle
Michael Maletta
Richard Malin
Bobby Malone
Paul Malone

Wes Manasco
Nick Mangan, *114*
George Manierre
Chuck March,* *126*
Larry Neal Marcus
Tom Markowski
Andy C. Marks
J. Michael Maroney
Hal Marret, *86*
Peter Martel
Alberto Martin
Edgar Martin
Gerald Martin
Jon W. Martin
Lester Martin
Mickey Martin, *67*
Richard Martin
Ernest Victor Martin, Jr.
Rene Martinez
Ken Mascarenas
Kevin Maslin
Jules Mason
Mark Mason
David Matheson
David Mathieson, *74*
John Mathieson
Le Wayne Matthews
Jerry Matus
David Lee Maulsby
David Lee Maulsy
Ed Mayberry
Jaye Mayhugh
David Maynard
Michael Houston
  McAdory, *77*
David McAlexander, *156*
Jerry McBride, *6*
Thomas Khamba
  McCardle
Tom McCardle
Palmer McCarter, *136*
Rosemary McCarthy
Alexander (Sandy)
  McClelland
Mark McCloskey
James McClure
Steve McCool
Larry McCoy
Roger McCoy
Roger McCraw
Jim McCreary, *125*

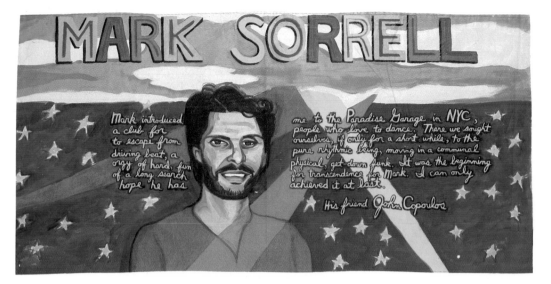

Curt McCullough
John W. McDonald, Jr.
Curt McDowell
Curt A. McDowell
Michael McDowell
William McDowell
Dennis McElhattan
Pat McGee
Wayne McGee
Kenneth McGowan, *126*
Robert McGrath
Ricky McKenzie
Stewart McKinney,* *103*
Michael McKinnon, *102*
Dennis McLain
Jake McLaughlin
Mac McLaughlin
Paul McLean
Bill McLeod
David McManus
Herman McNeill
Daniel Joseph McTague
Bill McTarnahan
Bob Meadows
Wendell Meek
Scott Meierding
Richard Meinhart, *73*
Peter Mejic
Mike Melig
Leonard Mengele
Bill Mercier

Hal Merritt
Zon Merritt
Mark Metcalf, *77*
Rod Meth
Allen Meyer
Gordon Meyer
Mundo Meza, *67, 125*
Steven J. Michalowski
Justin Mickler
John Middlebrook
Wayne Mielke
Aaron John Miller, *120*
Bill Miller
Chuck Miller
Court Miller, *101*
Gilbert Miller,* *85*
Glenn Miller, *123*
Henry Miller
John Miller
Martin Miller
Paul Miller
Paul B. Miller
Sam Miller
Stephen A. Miller
Francois Millet
Craig Alan Mills
James Mincey
Charlie Minehart
In Memory Of All
  Minnesota Victims of
  AIDS

John Minor
Michael Minor
John Mishler
Gary Mitchell
John Mitchell
Tommy Mitchell
William Mitchell
Al Mizner
Kevin Moberly
Ed Mock, *101*
Eddie Mohr
Poni Mon Dada
Eric Moniz
Gary L. Monroy
Roosevelt Montgomery
Bill Moon
Nolan Moon
Gary Moonert
Eric Moore
James Moore
Lawrence Moore
Randy Foster Moore
Victor Morales
Robert Morana
Wayne Morden
Miguel Morgado
Ron Morini
Chuck Morris, *26*
Don Morris
Ronald L. Morris

Thad Morrison
Jack Mort
Kyle Douglas Moses
Eric Mosley
David Mount
Leon Mouton
Rick Mowery
Johannes Mueller, *72*
John Mulhern
Richie Mullen
Layton Mullins, *57*
Mike Mumaw
Alex Murphy
Michael Murphy
Charles R. Musgrave
Jeff Mylett
Dan N.
Jack Natkin
Lorenzo Navarro
Paul Neesom
Bob Nelson
George Nelson
Richard Newton
Hugo Niehaus
Kenny Niles
Avi Nilson
Jon Nite
Norman Nomano
Jim Nordmeyer
David Norrie

Perry Norris
Curt Norrup
Gary Noss
Jay Nova
Gary Novack
Ramiro Nuñez
Ray Nyquist
Billy O.
Jim O'Connell
Michael O'Connor
Michael O'Leary
Pat O'Leary
Bill O'Malley
Sean O'Neil
Toby O'Neill
Tom Oates
Tommy Oates
Scott Oatman
Gene Oblander
Roger Obst
Victor Offenberg
Dennis Oglesby
Chris Olds
Joe Olea
Robert Oleksy, Jr.,* *13*
David Oleson
Jim Oliver
Patrick Oliver
Doug Olsen
Terry Omer
Louis Onesta
Jonathon Orrell
Phil Osborne
Lew Ostenink
Bill Ouellette
Dave "Bob" Owen
Walter Owen
J. P.
S. P.
Louis Pace
Chris Page
Tom Paille
Alan Paine
David Palmer
Michael Palmer
Rob Pambid
Tony Panico
Nick Paradisis, *116*
Nick Paris
Richard Paris,* *20*

Gerry Parker
Don Parkey
Jerry Parrott
Bob Parsons
Joseph Partlow
Randy Partlow
David Pasko
Neil Patchek, 61
Glenn Paul
Timothy Robinson Paul
Martin Pearl
Gerald Pearson
Jim Pearson
Jerry Peck
Richard Pelley, 117
Rene Pelliccia
Bubby Pennstrom
Robert Penny
John F. Pereira
Abel Perez
Joe Perry
Larry R. Perry
Stephen Perry
Steve Perry
Glenn Person
John Peterman
Bill Peters
Gene Peterson
Pete Peterson
Tony Pfafflin
Scott Pharis
Bob Phelps
Clyde Phelps, 76
Lloyd Phelps, 105
Mark Philips
Michael Pierce
Randy Pike
Morgan Pinney
Rafael Pinto
Lewis Pionke
Billy Piper
Kap Pischel
Perry Pittman
Thom Plemmons
Steven Plumlee
Terry Poe
Zanny Poelker
Woody Poland
John Politano,* 124
John Kuhner Ponyman

Bill Pope
Paul Popham
Douglas Porcaro
Roger Portal, 75
Ron Pouliot
Bill Powell
Carlton Powers
Mark Powers
Billy Prato
Chuck Preston
Jed Prewit
David Price
John Price
Jonathan Price
Elizabeth Prophet
Provincetown
    Anonymous
John Provost, 6
Herb Pruett
Ted Puckett
Christopher Puertas
Kurt Pulver
Sam Pumilia
Qia Qodrea
Stephen Quesada, 6
Steven Quesada
Ralph A. Quick
John Quinn
John Patrick Quinn, 89
José M. Quintaîlla
M. R.
Larry Rabbitt
Dennis R. Radabaugh
Keith Rahner
Richard Rajkawski
Anthony Ramirez
Gregorio Ramirez, 17
José Ramirez
William S. Randles, 134
Mike Reardon
Len Reber
Chuck Recob
Bobby Redfern
Carter T. Reed
Mike Reed
David Reeder
Fred Reeves
Randy Reichart,* 70
Alan Reid
Joel Reid

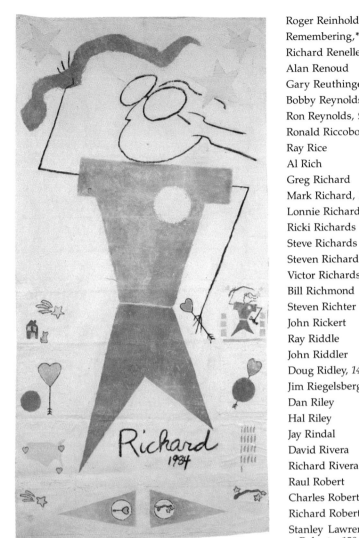

Roger Reinhold
Remembering,* 82
Richard Renelleman
Alan Renoud
Gary Reuthinger
Bobby Reynolds
Ron Reynolds, 97
Ronald Riccobono
Ray Rice
Al Rich
Greg Richard
Mark Richard, 115
Lonnie Richards
Ricki Richards
Steve Richards
Steven Richards
Victor Richardson
Bill Richmond
Steven Richter
John Rickert
Ray Riddle
John Riddler
Doug Ridley, 14
Jim Riegelsberger
Dan Riley
Hal Riley
Jay Rindal
David Rivera
Richard Rivera
Raul Robert
Charles Roberts
Richard Roberts
Stanley Lawrence
    Roberts, 150
Steve Roberts
Arnold Robinson
Curt Robinson
Manny Robinson
Clarence Robinson, 65
Norman Rockne
Jimmy Roddy
Paul Rodenkirch
Paul Matthew Rodenkirk
Mike Rodgers
Jeffrey Roger, 46
Joel Rogers
Susan Piracci Roggio
Paul Rohrer, 48
Norman Rollings
Warren Rollins

Charlie Romero
Rebel Wayne Romero
Richard Romo
Hugh Stuart Rondell
Al Rosen
Jeff Rosenfeld, 155
Bernard Roth
Rex Roundy
Michael Ruben
David Rude
Bruce Allan Rudolf
Randy Ruhlman
Dan Rundle
Frank Runnels
John Michael Rushing
Bruce Russell
James R. Russell
Livingston Russell
John Russo
Robert Rutledge
Marco Ruvalcaba, 112
Bill Ryan
Dennis Ryan,* 113
Hugh Ryan
Mark Ryan
Ric Ryan
Lee Rymer
Al S.
Bob S.
D. S., 156
David S.
Louis Sada
Mike Saddler
Don Saglin
Donald R. Saglin
Jose Salles
Bill Salmon
Victor Sanchez
Rock Sand
Dr. William A. Sandberg
Dean Sandmire
Richard Sanor
Paul Sansone
Daniel Sauchuk
Nancy Sawaya
Brad Sawtell
Alan Sawtelle, 39
Toby Scanland
James Scaramuzino
Gary Scarberry

Laura Schaffer
Mark Schatz, 126
George Scheeler
Jay Schelby
Rick Schlie, 89
Joe Schmall
Steve Schmidt
Bruce Schneider
Louis Schneider
Charles Schrader
Jim Schroeder, 77
Lee Schroyer
John Schubat
Bill Schultz
Bob Schultz
Tom Schumann
M. Robert Schwab
Robert Schwab
Bill Schwartz
Ron Schwert, M.D.
George Scognamillo
Dick Scott
Lloyd Elliot Scott
Robert "Scotty" Scott,* 113
Walfa Scott
David Scudder, 39
David Sears
Howard C. Sears
R. Kirk Seaton
Mario Sebastian
Michael Sebastian,* 20
John Selby
Rodney Sellers
Ryan Serrels, 112
Stephen Shapiro
Hank Sharp
Jerry Shatzer
Henry W. Shaver
Harold Shaw
Ric Shea
Corey Shearer, 117
Fred Shepler
Henry Shernoff
Jim Sherrick
Ron Sherrill
Greg Sherwin
Larry Shine
Marvin Shipley
Phillip Shippy
Willie Short, 61

James Brooke Shoulberg
Jim Shoulberg
James Ramsey Shrode
John Shubat
Sergei Shullski
Eric Shuman
Jon Shymansky
Dennis Sickler
James Siegel
Joe "Windburn" Sietz
John T. Siler
George Silkworth
Livio Silvestre
Jose Simon
Jon Sims
David Sindt,* 37
Charles Skipper
Michael Sklar, 16
Amy Sloan
Brice W. Small
André Smith
Bob Smith
Craig Smith
Donald R. Smith,* 20
Greg Smith,* 122
James Byron Smith
John D. Smith
Justin Smith
Louis Smith, 99
Marshall Smith
Michael Allen Smith
Pat Smith
Phillip Smith, 77
Robbie Smith
Willi Smith, 100
William C. Smith
Timmy Smithwick
Jim Snow
Bill Snyder
Chuck Solomon
Ricky Todd Solomon
Sydney & Jim Soons, 43
Mark Sorell
Mark Sorrell, 152
Ricardo Souza
Stan Spaeth
Bill Spalding
Jay Spears
Tommy Spotts
Michael Spurlock

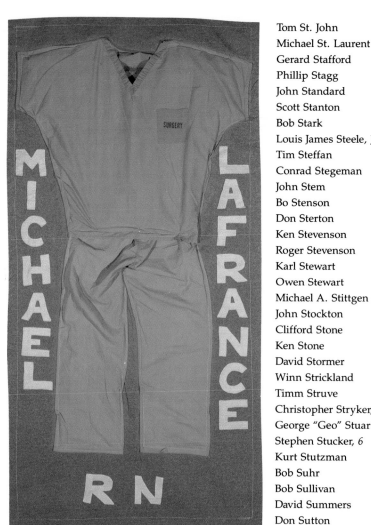

Michael LaFrance, an operating room nurse, worked at the same hospital as medical bookkeeper Ian Ferrar. "He was always more concerned about other people than himself," says Ian, who solicited help from his lover Bob Munk to sew this panel in Michael's honor.

Tom St. John
Michael St. Laurent
Gerard Stafford
Phillip Stagg
John Standard
Scott Stanton
Bob Stark
Louis James Steele, Jr.
Tim Steffan
Conrad Stegeman
John Stem
Bo Stenson
Don Sterton
Ken Stevenson
Roger Stevenson
Karl Stewart
Owen Stewart
Michael A. Stittgen
John Stockton
Clifford Stone
Ken Stone
David Stormer
Winn Strickland
Timm Struve
Christopher Stryker, 101
George "Geo" Stuart
Stephen Stucker, 6
Kurt Stutzman
Bob Suhr
Bob Sullivan
David Summers
Don Sutton
Patrick Sweeney, 112
Jim Swindel
Dennis T.
F. T.
T. T.
Ron C. Tacoma
Brian Tadesco
David James Taggart
Mickey Talbot
Michael Talbott
Bob Tananis
Tim Tasker
Bruce Richard Taylor
Tom C. Terrific
Sal Territo
Michael Thimmes
Dan Thomas
Garson Thomas

James Thomas
Joel Ken Thomas
Michael Thomas
Bobby Thompson
Charles Thompson
David Thompson
David R. Thompson, 62
Harvey Thompson
Larry David Thompson
Jerry Thornburg
Wayne Thornton, 74
To Those We Love and Lost
David Tibbits,* 113
Lorenzo (Larry) Ticol
Mark Tompson
Mitchell Toney
Juan Miguel Torres
Bob Torrey
Chip Torrez
Tony Torrise
Ken Towle
Ed Towne
Tony Trancoso, Jr.
Tony Trantrafil
Gar Traynor
Jack Tremaine
Tony Tripi
Ralph Troglione
Mark Trollan,* 95
John Trowbridge, 6
John Mott Trowbridge
Mark True
Richard Truelove
Mark Tsakirgis
Jerry Tubbs
Joseph Tucci, Jr.,* 58
J. T. Tucker
John Benjamin Tucker
John T. Tucker
Ray Tuite
Freddy Tuliper
Mark Turkel
Toby Tyler
Andrew Tzoumas
Unacknowledged AIDS Victims, 160
Baird Underhill, 94
Unknown,* 83
The Unknown Alone

Unknown But Not
  Forgotten
Bailey Upchurch
Chris Urbanik
Christopher Urbanik
Steven Uslander, *89*
Frank Uster
Kent Valentin
Todd Van Bortel
Johan Van Der Zwaan
Terry van Laarz, *133*
Steve Van Sant
Tom Van Strien
Dr. Rava Vara
Ernesto Vargas
Paul Varner
Gray Vasse
Mundy Vega
Felix Velarde-Muñoz
Ron Verducci
Carl Verzilli, Jr.
Russell Viera
Hank Vilas
Danny Villa
James "Jim" Vineyard
Rusty Virgen
Michael John Virhales
Gary Visage
Kenneth Vittatoe
Doug Vogeler
Martin Voigt
Douglas Von Lloyd
Paul Von Steinmann
Bill W.
C. E. W.
J. A. W.
Dr. Thomas Waddell, *87*
Gerd Wagener, *130*
David "Mike" Waits
Mel Wald
Jerry Walker
Paul Walker, *99*
Jac Wall, *53*
Corman Wallace
Mik Wallace
Gary Walsh
Anton Walter
David Walters
Jerry Walters
Barney Ward

Eddie Ward
Michael Ward
Bill Warren
Paul Watford
Billy Watkins
Bill Watson
Chaz Watson
George Watson
Michael Watton
Larry Waurin
Gary Way
Phillip Weathers
Troy Bud Webb
Stephen Weber
Steven Weber
Thom Weber
Tom Weber
Stephan Weddell
Mike Weed
Michael Weiland
Steve Weiner
Frank C. Weis
Henry Weitzer
Ronald P. West
Paul Wheeler
Tom Wheeler
Wayne Whitcomb
Bob White
Stuart White
Larry Whited
Gary Whiteley
Steve Whitfield
John Whittington
Ron Whitworth
Dale Widmark
Hugo Wiehaus, *89*
Bill Wike
Arthur Wilfield
Frank Wilkes
Ken Wilkes
Hank Will
Tom Willenbecher
Christine Williams, *42*
Cody Williams
Gene Williams
Rodney Williams
Sam Williams
Duane Willis
John Willis
Gary Wilson

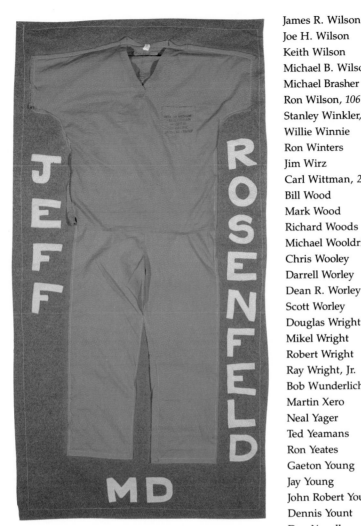

Ian Ferrar met Los Angeles pediatric physician Jeff Rosenfeld through Michael LaFrance. "They were best friends," says Ian. "And they were both giving people, right to the very end."

James R. Wilson
Joe H. Wilson
Keith Wilson
Michael B. Wilson
Michael Brasher Wilson
Ron Wilson, *106*
Stanley Winkler, *6*
Willie Winnie
Ron Winters
Jim Wirz
Carl Wittman, *20*
Bill Wood
Mark Wood
Richard Woods
Michael Wooldridge
Chris Wooley
Darrell Worley
Dean R. Worley
Scott Worley
Douglas Wright
Mikel Wright
Robert Wright
Ray Wright, Jr.
Bob Wunderlich
Martin Xero
Neal Yager
Ted Yeamans
Ron Yeates
Gaeton Young
Jay Young
John Robert Young
Dennis Yount
Don Yowell
Michael Z.
Richard Z.
Tony Z.
Tommy Zalewski
Mark Zambrano
John Zimarowski
Tony Zinni
Joe Zogby
Kit Zoll
Ignacio Zuazo
Gene Zuchelli
Larry Zullo

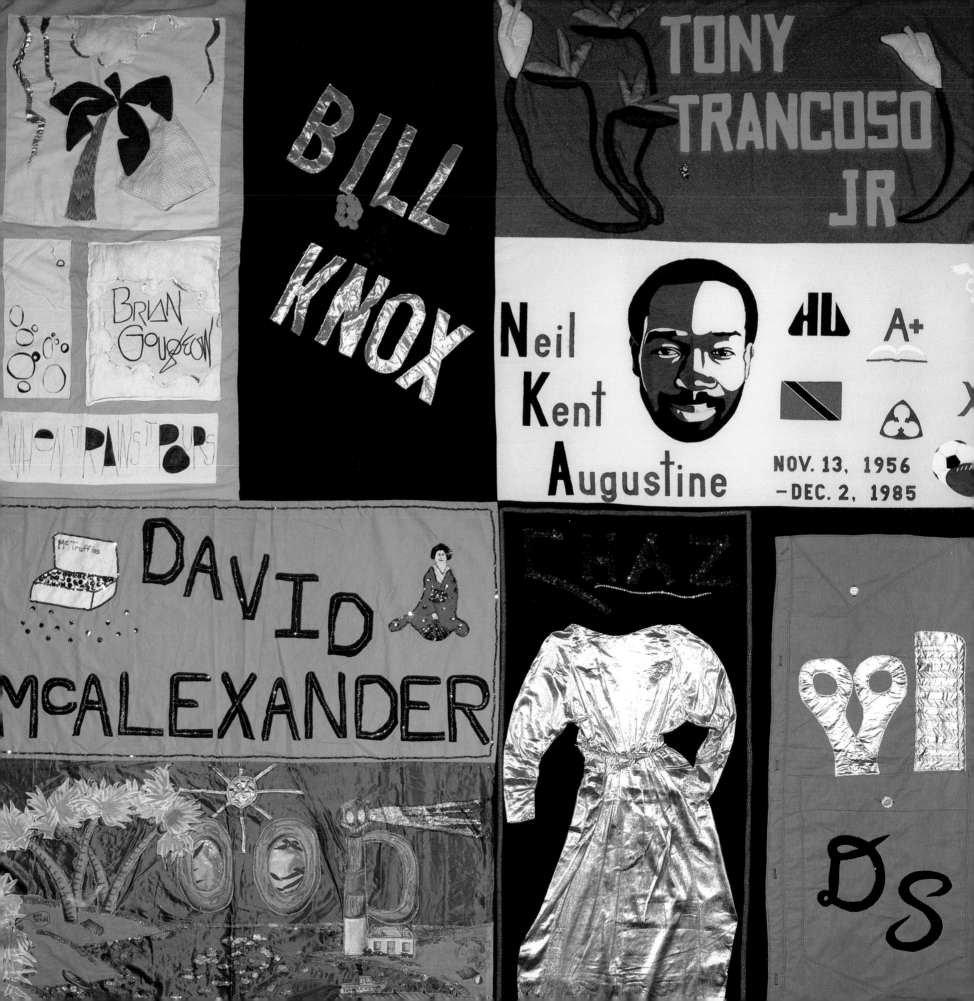

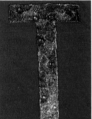he Quilt was created in homes across America by the families, friends and lovers of people lost to AIDS. While they represent a great diversity of people and backgrounds, they are united by their shared experience of a devastating epidemic.

For many Americans, the AIDS epidemic has become the tragedy of our generation, profoundly affecting every aspect of our lives. As a nation, we have struggled not only against a disease, but also against the equally destructive enemies of ignorance, hysteria and bigotry.

At times it seemed that we lacked the national will to conquer AIDS, and many of us despaired.

This quilt is a gift from the hands and hearts of thousands of Americans who have learned not to despair. It stands as a statement of hope and remembrance, a symbol of national unity and a promise of love.

Each of us at the Project has been deeply honored by the trust and touched by the love of the panel-makers. They and their loved ones — those who have fallen and those who remain — have become a part of our lives.

We will never forget them.

Cleve Jones
Executive Director

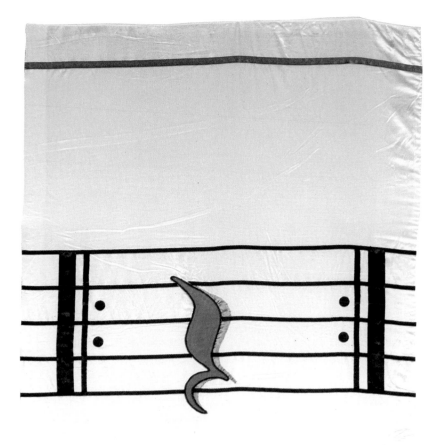

The NAMES Project wishes to express its gratitude to the following: Apple Computer, Design and Interior Furnishings Foundation for AIDS (DIFFA), Flying Tigers, Henry Calvin Fabrics, KPIX-TV, Neiman-Marcus, Office of Congresswoman Nancy Pelosi, Paramount Flag Company, *People* magazine, *San Francisco Examiner*, the U.S. National Park Service and the Westinghouse Broadcasting Corporation.

The author, photographer and designer especially wish to thank DC Typography, Eastman Kodak Company, Innervisions Studio, Kajun Graphics, The New Lab, David Karnes, Patricia Koren, Richard Lulenski, Marcia McGetrick, Richard Newberger, Esther Newberg, Michael Small, Bryan Smith, Laurie Smith and the photographers who donated their work: Tom Alleman, Peter Ansin, Marc Geller, Matt Herron and Paul Warchol.

We are greatly indebted to all the panel-makers who opened up their lives in long interviews, and regret that due to time and space restraints, we were unable to include all their stories in the book.

The staff and volunteers of The NAMES Project are particularly grateful for the friendship and support shown us by Pocket Books and Simon & Schuster: Bill Grose, Irwyn Applebaum, Pat Cool, Jack Romanos, Gina Centrello, Anne Maitland, Boris Mlawer, Jean Anne Rose and Kara Welsh.

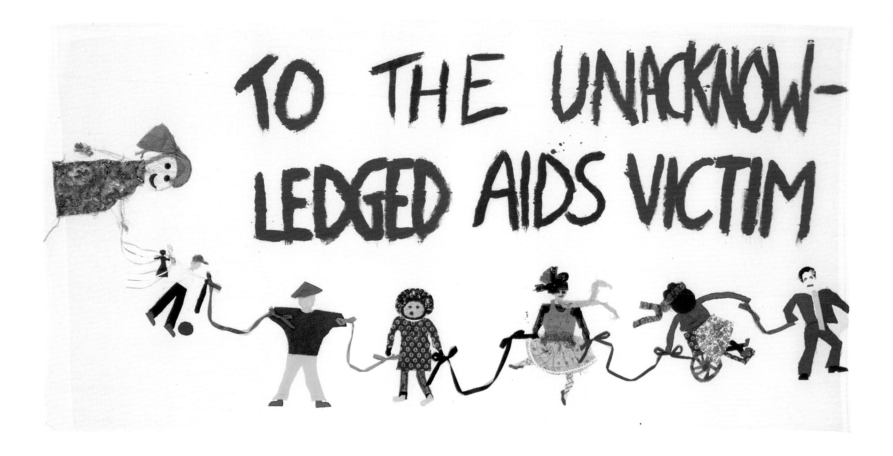

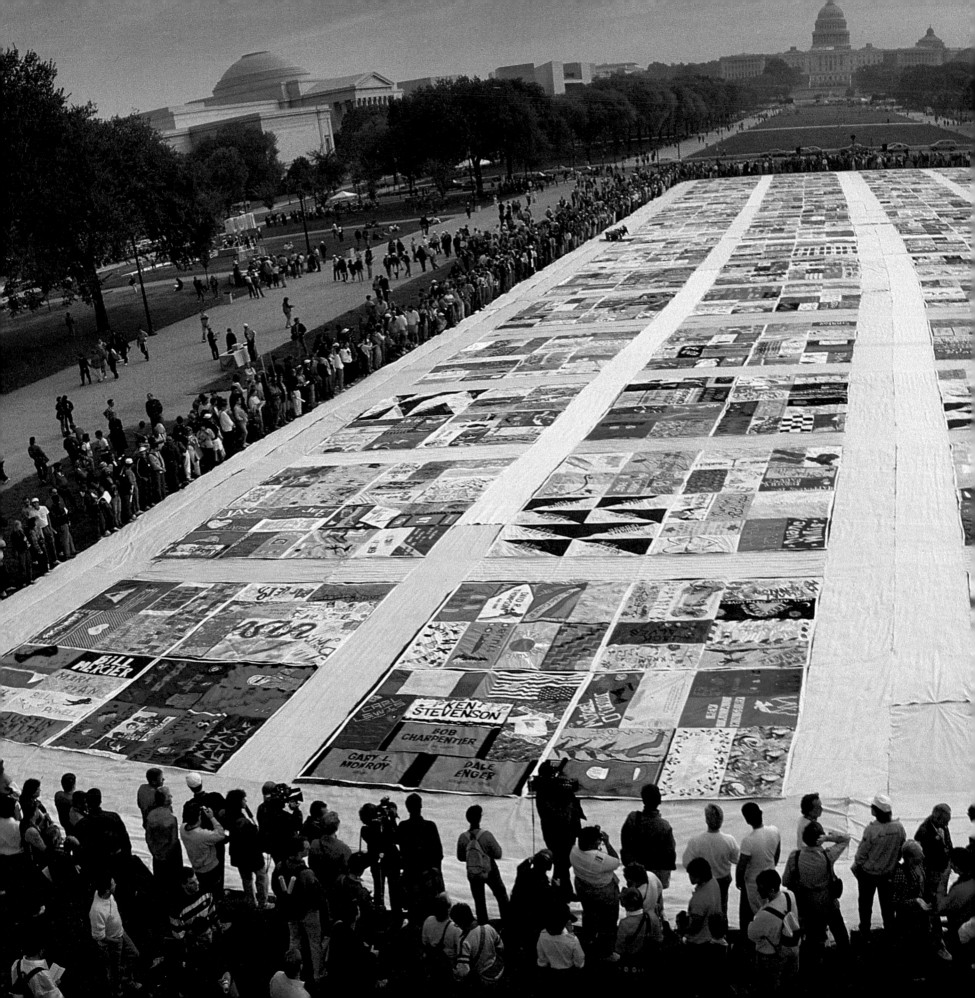